GU00976077

Cats Dogs and Wellies

(life as a city vet)

By Tim Roe

Published by Snowflake and the Egg

All illustrations by Sophie

Published by Snowflake and the Egg

323, Drayton High Rd.
Hellesdon, Norwich, Norfolk

Copyright. T.J.Roe   September 2005

Printed in Great Britain by

Hangar Press Limited, Oak St. Norwich.

ISBN 978-0-9551444-0-0

Acknowledgments

My family, for enduring support; and especially Sophie for coping with persistent pestering! My grateful thanks to Paul and Dan at Hangar Press in Norwich for making it all happen so easily.

This book can also be purchased:

1. via email, t.roe@netcom.co.uk
2. via the Willow Veterinary Clinic website, www.willow-veterinary-clinic.co.uk
3. and from the Willow Veterinary Clinic, 323 Drayton High Road, Hellesdon, Norwich NR5 6AA

Foreword

This book started to develop when I began to write a few articles in the last century about being 'the vetinary', but I soon realised that each week, each one added to a rapidly developing alternative diary. So, a seed of an idea, to produce a small book, became a definite maybe; and here it is, because so many people asked me to do it.

I kept writing the articles because I enjoyed it, and because it provided me with something to look back upon - I don't keep a diary!

I hope that these pages, containing a selection of short extracts from my musings during one day, a particular week; or even about a constant train of thought, will paint pictures for you! Pictures of my veterinary life in a busy companion animal practice in Norfolk - and how that life makes me 'tick'.

The people and animals are the true characters, but I also wish that the delightful line drawings by Sophie, at the very least, make you smile.

Vets can fly

Several years ago, a well-known and rather eccentric vet was severely reprimanded by our governing body, The Royal Veterinary College disciplinary committee, for conduct unbecoming to the profession and likely to bring all of us into some form of disrepute. His crime? To drink as much alcohol as possible and then take his single-seater fighter aircraft up to the heavens and spend several wild minutes dive-bombing local residents enjoying a quiet Sunday afternoon sailing off the south coast or topping up their tans!

Now call me 'old-fashioned', but this story made me laugh long and hard, despite the potential mortal danger that these episodes created. In fact, no one was damaged. 'Vetinary' survived, lost his pilot's licence, and received a short period helping 'Her Majesty' with her pleasure.

My experience of our profession is such that the above performance 'smacks' typically of the rather 'cavalier' attitude to life that some of us live and breathe - and it takes me nicely to a 'flying' episode that I experienced in my career.

It is one of the loveliest sights on this earth to watch the cattle on the marshlands of Norfolk, heads down, enjoying the rich grasses and looking the picture of health as the summer sun beats down on their shining coats - but come the end of the warmer months, many of those same beasts are herded into winter quarters for fattening. Their freedom is curtailed, and they face several months in the deep litter sheds.

They quickly accept their new homes, but the first day or two can be fraught with..... shall we say 'exuberance'! That natural freedom, being stifled, can lead to a lot of rushing around in the pens and negative response to humans.

Certain farms were notorious for 'Winter madness', mainly because their cattle lived the summer months on the most remote marshes and had little, if any, human contact!

I had to go to one such farm to examine a lame heifer within a group of twenty or so, held in a yard, and I immediately realised that this was to be a tricky assignment. The farmer, bless him, meant well, but his utterance of 'Whoa' at fairly regular intervals and waving his long stick, seemed to achieve little except to increase the speed at which the animals ran round the yard. It reminded me of a rodeo scene, but all taking place within a space the size of a tennis court.

Bravery surfaced and Roe stepped into the enclosure to 'sort' things, holding a lasso on the end of a long stick specifically placed to allow the charging beast to run headlong to capture - what a joke! These youngsters thought it was a special game and simply ran faster, beginning to 'donkey-kick' as they went past me.

What happened next feels just like a scene from Tom and Jerry, as one animal ran past very close to me, turning sharply, kicking out with its back legs on that turn. The tips of each hoof made contact with my waistbelt, and I was flipped up and into the air, flying about twelve feet backwards, hitting the wall of the yard about eight feet up and slumping unceremoniously to the ground where I sat wheezing for several minutes, in the throes of a severe winding.

On reflection, I was lucky to have lived! Avoiding massive injury by taking a step back as the heifer ran past, and being so badly winded that I was totally relaxed as I hit the wall; though severe bruising of body and pride followed and, by the way, the farmer refused to pay for the visit, seeing as I had failed to treat his beast!

Test flight one was over but more was to follow, as I struggled to enter the record books for the greatest 'animal-propelled flight' in history. More of that later.

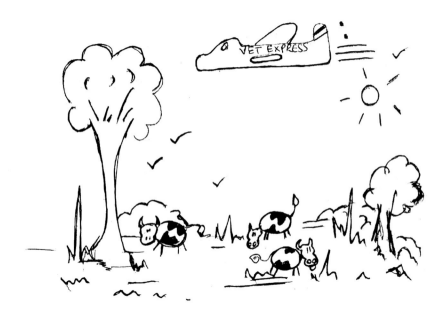

Porcupine sandwich

It has not been important to give my opinion upon the general state of captive animals during my career. Wildlife parks, zoos, and collections seem deemed to survive based upon public support.

We have a nation of discerning animal-lovers who are well-educated in the area of animal welfare, voting positively with their feet, so those good concerns will, and do continue to prosper because they have animal welfare, and species survival at heart.

I rather foolishly offered to visit one delightful zoo and gardens at the request of the curator, concerned with a female porcupine who appeared 'off colour'.

These were not small, cuddlesome beasties, but grumpy, aggressive ones, capable of confronting you with a three foot fan of ten-inch long spines, with vicious points and 'quick-release' facility for sticking them in anyone, or thing, that upset them.

The problem was not the sick female, but her very protective, even larger male partner, who paced up and down behind the keeper and I, fended off by a bristly broom, wielded by keeper number two.

The plot thickens!...The female had been in season just recently: in fact, the week before, and the diagnosis that I made of a womb infection from six feet away was, to my mind, inspired!

The next hurdle!...How to inject an animal with antibiotics, who is nine-tenths prickles?

A large sack saved the day, being rapidly thrown over her, flattening the spines, and aiding the keeper in wrestling her to a standstill, allowing me to make my move with syringe full of penicillin...Well, that was the plan!

The large August crowd that had gathered (snapping pictures, and giggling over my predicament) saw it all happening before I did. I turned to smile, triumphantly, but as I knelt beside the female, a torrent of yells and guffaws came simultaneously from behind. From the corner of my eye, I caught sight of the rapidly charging male, who, having eluded his keeper, was making straight for me, head down, spines flexed!

I tried to climb to my feet, slipped on the damp grass, and fell prey to the males advances. Cameras flashed; the laughter grew to uncontrolled uproar. The male made as if to launch himself, then stopped very suddenly, immediately sniffed my right leg, and began to make 'porcupine love' to my wellington boot, as I desperately tried to extract my leg. Every available camera began to flash and click.

Eventually I escaped and hopped to the perimeter fence, to tumultuous applause, taking a bow into the bargain, though I found out later, on inspection of the wellington with 'sex appeal' that the female had urinated all over both boots, and that in her present state, this was an aphrodisiac to the frustrated chap.

So back to my original topic of zoos etcetera. We have some lovely collections, of excellent quality in Norfolk, and having worked in several of them, I feel able to say that they show the highest level of animal care. This is so frequently shown by the animals being in good condition, and living in well-maintained surroundings.

Animal exhibits will not go away, so I feel that we should all support those good ones, and report the bad examples, so that standards are always looking to be maintained and improved.

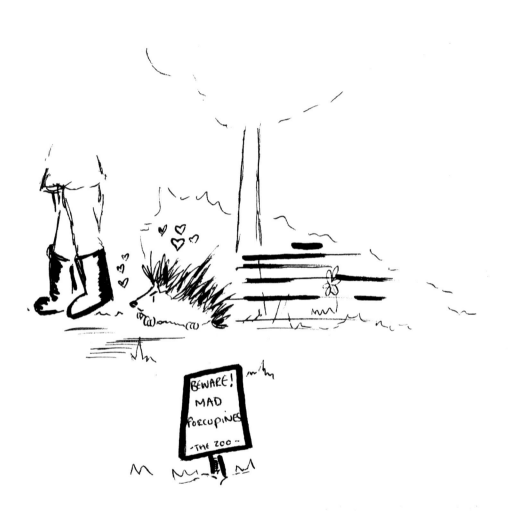

4

Sidney's common sense

It will not be apparent instantly, that you have a new correspondent this week! The 'two-legs' have gone away, so I've grabbed this opportunity to get a few things down on paper, and set the record straight. I've tried the keyboard on the piano - four hands work really well! and I play good tunes, so the computer should be easier - just jump around on it and press 'spellcheck' to make it understandable.

They've stuck me in a kennel for three days, and expect me to sit here patiently, with no carpet to chew, no rugs to run under and scrumple up into a ball, and no furniture to get my claws into. How an earth is a chap expected to express himself?

Anyway, here are a few thoughts from Sidney Roe, youngest feline member of the Roe household, mainly to get my own back about being left locked up (all safely, they said) but also because I was reading some of the silly stuff in the paper basket last week; do you know that newspapers make cracking scent-marking posts, as long as the 'two-legs' don't tidy them up too often!

So, I was reading that we now have more computers in our homes than pets - more than 7.8 million of those 'wizzy-whirry' things.Well, they don't taste and don't smell, and I can't see where those flying windows come from. I've sat for hours, hiding behind the screen, regularly pouncing out to catch one, and missed every time.They don't play with you either - so get a new pet instead!

In one of the papers, it said that we are pampering our pets too much, destroying their health with expensive food and making us fat!…Well, I like being fat. My fat belly helps me to roll around more successfully, and the food is really good, because the 'two-legs' with the long blonde hair, secretly feeds me some really smelly, tasty stuff from a tin when the grumpy 'two-leg', who never spoils me,(and works in the funny-smelling place they all call Willow Vet Clinic) isn't there.

He reckons that it makes me fat, but I showed him the other day, when he complained about 'us cats' being spoiled too often - I brought a dead pigeon into the house and spread feathers everywhere…It was great, because I know that all the other 'two-legs' hate that sort of mess, and make him clear it up! Then, they feed me more, because they think it will stop me doing that sort of thing. They didn't realize that I just found the pigeon lying around in the garden.

In another paper, it said that pet owners are ruining the social behaviour and natural activity of domestic pets by keeping them isolated from pack or group interaction, without exercise or socialisation. And, by neutering them, breaking the normal processes of development and psychological expression!… What a load of twaddle! I like being neutered. All the cats I know that aren't are really bad-tempered, more often than not. They don't like playing around and you can't rely on them to turn up. They pee everywhere, and then argue about who owns where they peed… No! I can't get on with them. I prefer all my neutered mates at home, but that William is a bit 'stand-offish'.The 'two-legs' say that's because he only lives here part time. I'm sure that he's a proper 'Casanova', because he wanders off down the road, returning a few days later, smelling of cheap perfume, and needing a jolly good rest - sounds like fun! I might try that at some point.

Well, I'd better go just now. A nurse is coming to feed me, cuddle me and generally try to make me feel good. I suppose someone has to suffer in this way - It might as well be me! I may write again when 'old grumpy two-legs' is away next time, but until then, you'll just have to read his small offerings! I'll just sit here and wait.

Affectionately yours, Sidney kitten.

5

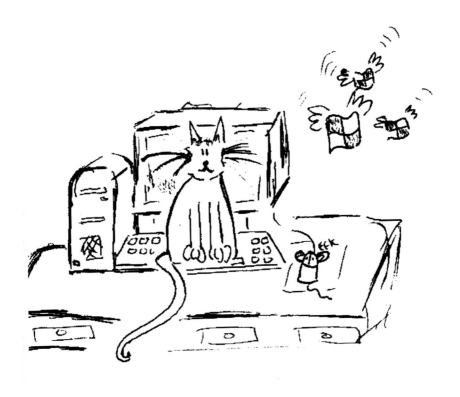

A little spot of Blarney

What I really wanted from Lisa, the seventh daughter of a seventh daughter - hence being imbued with the ability to read your palm, foretell your future, and relieve you of fifty pounds for a seven year game plan, was how would I enjoy my holiday in Ireland? And was I going to get a rest from the cares and concerns of a busy vet's life?

But Lisa told me more than that! And rather surprised me with her accuracy and foresight. It seemed that this little old lady, plying her trade in a cosy little caravan, a stone throw from the quayside of the lovely seaside town of Bantry, was going to prove that to my wife and children (who had already been to see her) that she had an uncanny ability to see into your past and predict something of the future.

I should have foretold that the Roe family could not go on their 'hols' without plenty of animal activity. Perhaps the little town close to the mountains where our holiday home was perched being called Ballylickey should have forewarned me.

You see the children of a vet think that you are 'on call' twenty four hours a day, even when on holiday. So youngest daughter spent a considerable part of the drive from Rosslaire advising me that sheep, that were either lying down (or were actually plastic bags, falsely accused of being sheep) were in need of my attention.

The whole family regularly shouted advice about avoiding the numerous little dogs that seem to roam the streets of all Irish villages at all times, seemingly certain of where they are going, but needing to run or walk down the middle of the road to achieve this.

When we arrived at our isolated holiday house, which was genuinely up a mountain, with no apparent neighbours for miles around, I was unloading the car, when, from nowhere a little Pomeranian dog appeared, who walked up to me confidently, sniffed my leg, walked away to the front gate, turned round to face me and while eyeballing me, cocked his leg. Was this an Irish greeting or a nosey neighbour? It was indeed the latter, because two days later, I found a jack russell terrier in the garden, who trundled away up the track, having cocked his leg up the wheel of my car.

I still don't know where they came from or where they went, but the old cat who walked past the french doors on Wednesday night obviously knew why he had come. You see the cry of, "Poor little thing" should have warned me of what was to come. I found my family round the side of the house with a tin of gourmet cat food, obviously purchased behind my back, secretively feeding the old moggy, who was, I'm sure, grinning all the way to Blarney.

"I suppose you thought raiding the bin wasn't good enough?" I asked the old Tom. "Should I bring a supply of food from the clinic for you next year?"

By the way, the whole week was interspersed with phone calls back home, regarding the well being of a 7 day-old kitten, wisely adopted by my eldest daughter the day before we went on holiday. Woodland Cat Rescue came to the rescue, and more of this next week... unless of course, any of you knew that already?

P.S.- I might have to leave Norwich one day. The attraction of the hand-written note in the window of the veterinary surgery in Castletownshend read 'Murphy's the Vets – gone out!' What a compelling title and reason for being shut! Only bettered by the road sign on one of the many steep hills found during our travels. As we turned a sharp corner it said "SLOW", painted on the road. A hundred yards further on, on the next corner was written, "SLOWER".

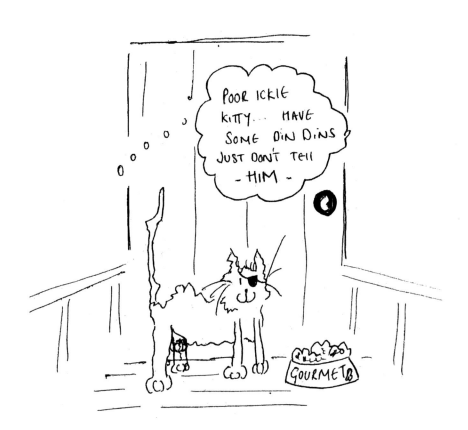

The kitten brought in from the cold

Weighing in at 150 grammes: wet, cold, and left stranded in the middle of a lawn wasn't a good start, but at least this little kitten was found before that cold and wet ended its life.

She was taken to Woodland Cat Rescue and subsequently to the clinic, where a full check up revealed little more than a very hungry and lost little soul, probably left behind by an inexperienced mum moving her litter to a new hiding place.

It was love at first sight, especially for my eldest daughter, who had to have her! I had no choice! She had to look after this small weanling, with eyes that were not even open, and who would need feeding every 2-3 hours. Did she realise that the rest of her summer holidays would be consumed by caring for this kitten?

Of course she did! The regime began of training this tiny cat to feed on milk replacer from a syringe and a plastic teat; alarms were set for wake up at 3 am and 6 am, and eldest child was firmly warned that I was only to be woken in an emergency - this was her baby!

That was two weeks ago, and now this little mite weighs in at 400grammes. She demands twenty millilitres of milk at each feed and has begun to show all the characteristics of kittens, which we love so much. Her little, wobbly legs are strong enough for an occasional stab at a pounce; she purrs like a traction engine and even showed signs of an early sidewind this afternoon.

She has consumed us all with her desire to survive, even beginning to show a little bit of temper when she doesn't get things her way, including coming everywhere with us; even on a family trip to a local restaurant last night, where our meal was interrupted by her requisite feeding time. She is adored by everybody she comes across and is presented to all our friends and family, who accept that this is quite normal Roe family behaviour. Of course it's reasonable to turn up at Sunday lunch with a basket containing kitten and bedding, plus a bag full of feeding equipment and a flask of warm kitten milk-replacer - people do this all the time!

So another little life has been saved, but as mentioned last week (as the carers at Woodland looked after her while we were away on holiday, bless them), little did we realise that they were backwards and forwards to the clinic nearly every day, trying to get her through a very tough first week, while steadfastly assuring my daughter that everything was ok when she rang to check on her progress.

Of course, she needed a name. It took five seconds to christen her 'Jelly bean' or 'jb' for brevity. She has even had a request played for her on radio Norfolk which I'm sure made her little fat head swell a just that little bit more.

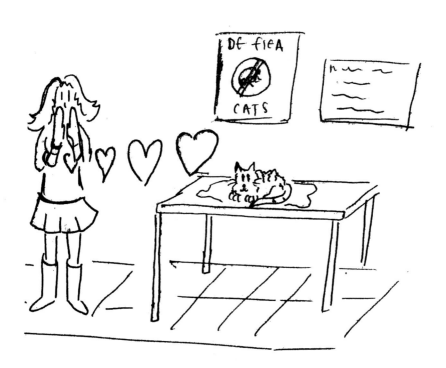

The trouble with a kitten is THAT Eventually it becomes a CAT

I have received so many comments and enquiries about the progress of our new kitten, Jelly Bean (or Jelly Five Bellies, as I have christened her), that I felt compelled to report on developments this week, leaving my usual clinic stories on the back boiler.

It has been quite marvellous watching this little thing develop. It's almost like seeing your own child grow up, learning new skills: walking, running, talking etc., but all compressed into a few weeks, instead of years - though some of her antics have a level of unacceptability.

Take for example, her toilet training, which at present has a zero rating. This kitten could pee for England. The copious amounts and 'mains pressure' facility is stupendous. The other evening I was holding her while introducing her to flying lessons. As she came into land on my chest, the flood gates opened. She drenched the front of my shirt, and continued as I held her out at arms length, until she had splattered an area a foot square on the parquet floor. She only weighs 450 grammes, but I'm sure that she delivered a continuous torrent for at least fifteen seconds, hence, I spent the next day comparing her to a Scottish spate river.

We won't go into the further complexities on number 'ones' and 'twos', but suffice to say, she has no concept of time or place - the world is her toilet!

Every aspect of her life brings laughter and joy to our family. Feeding time is particularly funny: being so demanding has forced us to try and wean her quickly, so she has been presented with solid food from three weeks onwards. Her little performance involves her food ending up like a paddy field, as she stomps around, pushing the food into little piles, which she then appears to suck up, with small 'squish' noises. Inevitably, it ends up all over her face, feet, and frequently in her ears; but she does avail herself of a wet cloth to wipe the excess away, and only because she can't move when full of a mixture of kitten food and milk!

Perhaps our greatest laughter results from her antics while playing: games from 'Bite the big toe' to 'Roly-poly kick boxing' are becoming common place. While the accuracy of the attack and the stealth with which it is made is improving all the time, she still miscues regularly enough, rushing away headlong into a chair as she makes her escape or falling over when she forgets to remember that you need at least four legs to make a quick getaway. You see her little 'bod' is still so soft and bendy that her fat pendulous stomach unbalances her whenever she tries to do something rapidly. Take for example the 'kamikaze' attack, where she pelts at full speed and jumps on your foot, chomping on fresh meat - the getaway is often flawed, because in an attempt to turn, get all four legs moving in the right direction, and inflict as much pain as possible for as long as it takes, something has to give. She either trips over her own legs or forgets to stop biting you, or escapes by running up your leg - a bad move, noticed rapidly and responded to by jumping headlong into oblivion. Luckily, she bounces well, then rushes somewhere to safety, reappearing within minutes for more! Life is so much fun.

I could go on forever! Try it - get your own kitten! It could seriously improve your health!

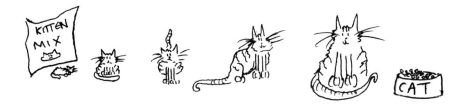

Taking a break

It was 11pm, Sunday 12th July. 'Vetinary' and family were on holiday in France, in a tiny fishing village called Batz Sur-Mer - just down the road from La Baule, where the England team stayed during the world cup.

On our kitchen wall was written 'Beckham was here' - hardly relevant as the church bells were ringing, horns hooting, shouts of 'Vive la France' - trois-zero, and all that!

We couldn't get away from it, and honestly, the good-natured exuberance of the locals was a pleasure to behold...

So, where are we going this week, I hear you ask? Well, like the football, which we were unable to avoid, our holiday showed that a vet cannot seem to get away from the job! I found myself scrutinising all the cats and dogs on the drive down from Cherbourg; and interestingly enough, during a five hour journey, I saw only three dogs. In Rennes, a very un-french looking little terrier, with a very french, wizened old lady, dressed in black; a quizzical collie outside the police station in Redon, and a very furry beastie, called a bouvier des flandres (this is a dog, by the way) as we arrived near to the coast, sitting in trance-like state on the steps of a house where a sign read 'Danielle and Phillipe, Astrology and Tarot readings'

This does not count my children crying for help at Mont St-Michel, where a black string vanished into a small dyke. They investigated, cried 'help', and I turned into 'vetinary-mode', only to find a cat on its holidays, attached by a harness to the black string and sitting on the bank of the dyke eating a sardine for lunch.

The owners appeared from the van, glared at our interference, as if to say 'Why can't we bring our cat on holiday, and keep it safely attached to a safety harness by a very safe piece of nylon cord?'

I was summoned again, as we passed through Pontchateau. Eldest child was concerned with the nasty brown stain around the eyes of a labrador sitting in the back of a nearby car! 'Probably entropion,' I explained (an eye condition where in-turning of the eyelids irritates the surface of the eyeball).

You see I was on holiday, but circumstance prevented me from complete anonymity from the job. Yet, I was still concerned that my research was not showing up many pets to look at during our car journey.

The next day, I tried to pay special attention, eventually finding out why so few had been visible...... **The answer?** They had all gone to the seaside. At Pouliguen, every conceivable dog on the western seaboard of France was out for the day: some poodles, but mainly little whizzing cross-breds, and portly labradors. I was a bit concerned for a little jack-russell, who seemed to have a bit of a flea-bite allergy, but the appearance of the owners concerned me more, so I kept out of it. Not that my french equates to an in-depth discussion about fleas!

It was a bit worrying, still casting my vet eye over pets, in a foreign country, where they would probably prefer me not to. Yet it shows that you can't switch off – anyway, free wine and food was being offered in the town square. Remember, France had just won the football World Cup. Oh well! 'Vive la France', if necessary. I suppose every cloud has a silver lining.

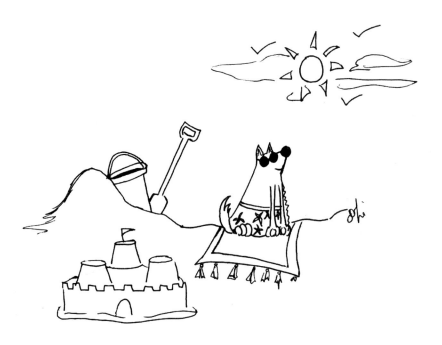

Only Down under!

It's an amazing thing that as vets we see a large variety of animals, as well as the diversity of disease that afflicts each species. Added to which, there is a huge assortment of creepy-crawlies that live on, or within, each species.

We have all manner of techniques and drugs to treat illness, and goodies which sort out those horrible parasites, but this week has been a real 'eye-opener' for me!

You see, our locum from Australia, Ian McBride, has been comparing and contrasting a vet's life in 'Oz' with mine; and it's jolly interesting, because at the start of the week I asked him to give me the most important differences that immediately came to mind, and he had little difficulty in launching into his 'top ten'.

He first explained that our perceived summer flea problem is a ripple compared to their tidal-wave. Apparently, the fleas are bigger, nastier and far more persistent than their 'country cousins' over here, and - wait for it! Many vets employ a 'flea wagon', which travels around the neighbourhood, towing a special bath, allowing owners to pop out into the street and pay a few dollars to have their dog bathed with an insecticidal wash to kill the offending parasites.

Now this conjured up all manner of images, but I was assured that it is a very professional service, used by many clients, and that it also helps to prevent another heinous parasite which we also have to deal with. The tick! Which is (most commonly) a nuisance for pets in Britain, but frequently causes a rapid, fatal paralysis in dogs in Australia.

He went on to explain that although gut upsets are a very common disease in our pets, we see nowhere near the level that they do, because out there, most dogs are kept outside, and are nearly all fed moist, tinned food, which, in their climate, can rapidly deteriorate, causing food-poisoning.

As the Australian client rushes to the vet to get treatment for all these 'nasties' they are also burdened by the fact that very few of them take out pet health insurance, hence it is sometimes a more difficult job for them to finance expensive pet treatment, perhaps influenced by the fact that you have to have a dog licence 'down-under'. But it's much cheaper to buy one if your pet is neutered! (what an excellent idea to help prevent unwanted litters etc).

So, dear readers, watch out if you are on your way to the southern hemisphere, where things that might be associated with your pet, and which bite, inject, and perhaps eat you, are bigger, uglier and more likely to do one of those things - or so I thought, until Ian assured me that it's not all that bad, and the facts about man-eating sharks, funnel-web spiders and snakes that hide in the toilet to attack you from the rear are grossly exaggerated.

If you want my opinion, I think all these stories are sent to us to prevent us all trolling off to their lovely country, and spoiling it for them. Thanks for the truth, Ian!

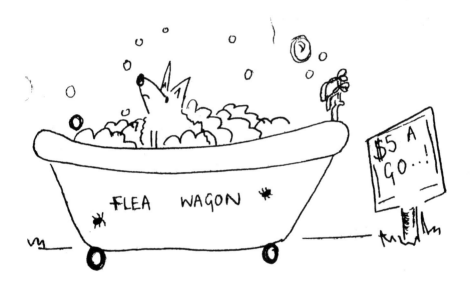

What's in a name ?

A pair of cats, called One and Two; dogs called Fairfax Frog and Vicar; a parrot called Perch – some of the myriad of amazing pet names I have come across in the past few years, and a subject of intense personal interest and pleasure. Why do we give such names to our pets?

Several years ago a client brought an oriental cat in for examination, whose name was 'Aka'. I of course, made the connection immediately.

'I suppose you named him after the famous clarinet player, Acker Bilk.'

'No!' she sneered. 'After the nomadic tribe called 'The Aka',' she continued.

Vetinary was firmly put in his place!

But, like a persistent puppy, I continue to tease, laugh and express surprise over the names chosen by owners for their pets. Their ingenuity is such a source of pleasure

I was talking to someone, just the other day, asking him why he had called his two tinkerish, ginger and white cats, Vic and Bob.

He replied that the kittens, when taken home at eight weeks had virtually chosen the names themselves, because they just sat there, taking swipes at each other for the the first hour, reminding him of the famous comedy pairing, bashing each other with rubber saucepans.

Unprompted, he continued, relating the progress of these little cats to local mobster-like status. Apparently, the five cats who lived next door were regularly terrorised by this pairing, who have learned to work together, mugging unsuspicious victims at any opportunity, and purely for fun!

Then he explained their relentless victimisation of the dog who lives a couple of doors down the road: Bob entices him out of his garden, along the road and round the corner, pretending to be a catchable cat, while Vic lies in wait, sitting on the wall just round that corner, from where he drops directly onto the dog's head! Bob, meanwhile rushes round to the other end and plants a set of teeth into its tail; then they both escape at speed to a safe distance, obviously, to laugh at the poor, bemused dog!

I was spell bound at the image of these two hoodlums, reeking havoc in their neighbourhood – and so aptly named!

Sometimes, it's the spur of the moment, as with Vic and Bob, or it might be something deeper? Not long ago, an owner came to reception to register his and his doberman's arrival. I asked if I could take the name, to which I received the gruff rejoin, 'Satan'!

I could not help myself. I looked him firmly in the eye and asked, 'Is that Mister or Miss ? '

Finally, I ask you to consider one vital ingredient of naming your pet! Can you genuinely stand on your doorstep at night, with the neighbours cooking their barbecue and shout, 'Stop messing about in the bushes, Vicar !' or 'Come on in Satan, mummy has prepared some lovely fresh meat for you!'... It bears thinking about!

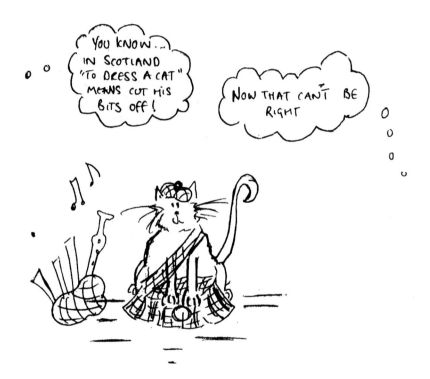

18

Strange things inside your pet

I have removed some amazing articles from domestic pets. Many of them from places that require major surgery to retrieve them, and most to the surprise and relief of their owners. But certain instances are so bizarre that they stay with you, in memory forever.

While working in Sunderland, a popular client rushed in one day, almost screaming that her pet retriever had swallowed one of her sheepskin gloves, yet his demeanour showed nothing other than huge pleasure for his achievement.

We radiographed his stomach, and behold, the shadow cast by five fat digits betrayed the presence of the glove in said stomach. The surgery that followed produced that rather sad glove, proudly presented to the owner. She was happy! While the pet felt sorry for himself.

Two days later, the same client rushed in, panic-stricken, 'He's swallowed the other one!' she cried.

'Are you sure?'

'Yes, I was holding it until he grabbed my finger as well. Then he gulped, and it was gone.'

'And he hasn't left your sight since then?'

'No, I brought him straight down to you!'

I quickly prepared him for a further operation. Then using the same incision site, I went to search for the second glove, chuckling at the irony of the situation. I opened up the stomach, and to my horror found... nothing! No glove! Not even a shred of sheepskin. It had vanished.

I phoned the owner. They assured me that they had seen it swallowed, and that the dog had not left their sight - but to this day I have no idea of the whereabouts of that second glove, and the owners never saw it again!

By the way, the dog survived his ordeal but took to swallowing pebbles from the beach. Luckily, he didn't require an operation to remove those foreign bodies, but many pets do!

I remember a couple of weeks back visiting a german shepherd dog that the owner reported as: putting on weight, being sick and making knocking noises.

As I felt the dog's abdomen it became clear that there was indeed a strange knocking noise, which began as I pressed on his stomach, causing him to turn round and stare intensely at his flank. As I pressed harder I could feel all manner of hard objects grating together. In short, on opening up his stomach I found thirty two pebbles from the beach, weighing one pound eleven ounces and obviously eaten because... Well, I don't know why he ate them! They don't taste nice or do anything valuable for a dog whatsoever! But this big chap found life unacceptable without thirty two stones in his stomach.

It refers me back to my comments a few weeks ago about not moralising about your pet's behaviour, because there is often no human equivalent. But that does not stand up to the test when compared to the poor human soul whose stomach and contents were gloriously displayed in the human pathology department at my university. He swallowed every piece of cutlery he could lay his hands on; for no apparent reason too. Perhaps the fact that he was displayed there suggested that he fared a little less happily than the dog.

Next week I will finish this section on the curse of the foreign body with perhaps the funniest, but at the same time the saddest case I have had to deal with when removing strange objects from a pet.

19

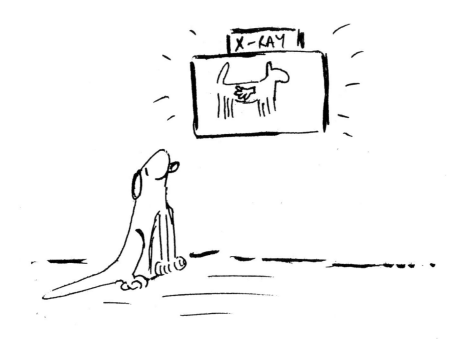

Sometimes we cannot help!

The surprise was that a ten week old puppy had swallowed a six inch long, solid, unbreakable, unchewable bone in the first place. But there he was, wagging his little labrador-tail for all he was worth, as I manipulated the bone in his stomach, this way and that, marvelling at his capacity, and desire, to swallow this relatively enormous, chewy plaything called a 'Nylobone'.

I had visions of him trying to ingest it, rather as a sword swallower might, sitting with his head held high for an eternity, as this large object was slowly consumed to its goal. We all smiled. The little chap was swiftly anaesthetised. The bone was removed safely; and twenty four hours later he was sent home, with advice to avoid leaving anything around for him to eat, except his food.

Exactly three days later, an astonished owner reported that the puppy had just swallowed the garage keys (which also included the car keys). Now, we were not talking small objects here. In fact, the x-ray showed eight keys, the largest of which measured just over six inches.

As for pup? He could not have been happier. A stomach full of metal, and ready for anything .

It was not quite 'all smiles' this time. I discussed the severity of such a problem-puppy with the owners, who agreed to surgical intervention this time, but felt almost unable to control this 'madcap' little fellow, who just grabbed any loose object, and tried to swallow it.

The keys were retrieved from the same place; puppy was sent home. But he only lasted eight days before he was brought back, wriggling and squiggling as before, delighted by all the attention, but with a stomach full again with foreign objects, including the keys, once again!

The sad result was that the owners could cope no longer, and after long discussion, they requested that the puppy should be put to sleep - and what a painful decision that was!

Please try not to be too judgmental about this decision! Dogs which behave in this way continue to behave in such a manner into later life, and eventually surgery is impossible due to the trauma caused by several operations, or one of the foreign bodies causes a painful death.

The amazing fact about this final swallowing episode was that along with the keys I removed the following: two pieces of wood, three stones, a Macdonald's happy meal toy, a doorstop, a plastic lid, a small bouncy ball; and (still to my amazement) a piece of window glass three inches long and just over an inch wide! How he managed all these objects remains a constant mystery, but it serves as a constant warning to all owners, as well as vets, that young dogs can decide to eat the strangest of objects, which can lead to heartache for everyone.

We were lucky when one of our pups demolished the egg basket, and about twenty eggs as well. He almost floated because he blew up with gas, and passed the most unusual 'scrambled egg' for the next few days… So, be warned!

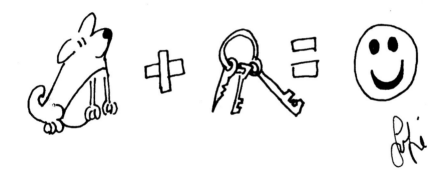

Bernard, Bodger, Birnham and Bulla

You know that something regularly catches my eye each week, as I look for a subject to write about. So it didn't seem strange to find that the letter 'B' appeared in many place, as I wound my way through yet another busy few days.

My diary starts with 'B' for Bernard. The name of a family I visited at the start of the week in a beautiful Scottish border village called Clovenfords, where they reside in a glorious historic mansion, once owned by Sir Walter Scott, called Ashiestiel, nestling in a farming estate on the banks of the River Tweed.

A few days off?... No such thing! I was surrounded by a myriad of lurchers and their crosses, who live 'Riley-like' in the house, and love a scratch from anyone who is willing. Inevitably, talk quickly turned to 'shop'. I'd espied one flea and was desperate to avoid deemed annoyingly helpful.

I tried to stay neutral for two blissful days, and gently indifferent, thinking that taking no side would be the best bet but, as usual, I let myself be drawn into giving an opinion on what was the best thing to use to kill these annoying pests.

As I left, having signed the visitors book, I wondered whether the great Sir Walter himself would have had any concern over the diminutive fleas affecting his dogs, surmising that he was probably more concerned with the human ones biting him.

'B' is for Bodger, a 'staffie' who delighted me with his described outrage at finding himself 'in the drink' so to speak while on a narrow boat holiday with his owners. Having fallen asleep on deck, he had gently slid towards the gunwales as the boat yawed, and onwards uceremoniously into the water, awakening rapidly, taking no harm - but collecting a very dented ego. His owners reported a thick atmosphere of indignancy from dear old Bodger for a considerable period after his dunking.

'B' begins the word 'Birnham', which describes a breed of cat owned by a dear lady who rang the practice today. She obviously means Birman but insisted on using her own term. Sheridan's Mrs Malaprop lives!...In Norwich.

And finally 'B' is for Bulla, the name of a boney, hollow prominence either side of a mammal's skull which houses the internal mechanisms linking the external ear via the eardrum to the brain.

It becomes infected in association with chronic ear disease, particularly in dogs, requiring very specialised, time-consuming surgery to put things right. And although it's happily not a common procedure, I've found myself carrying out this operation twice in the last week, compared to once in the previous year. Quite how fate arrives in this way, I'm unsure.

Bbbbbbbusy week?... I should say so!

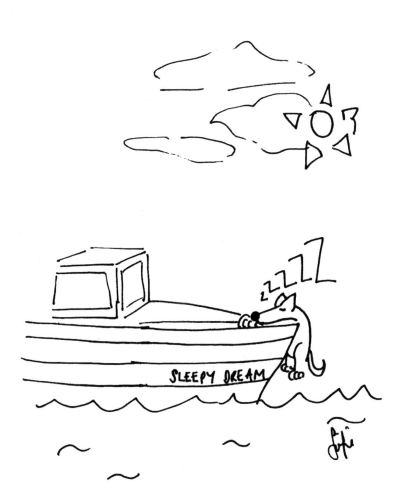

Toby does his stuff

Sometimes it is just impossible to separate personal feelings from the harsh reality of the job because I, like most of you, suffer the same emotions as other humans and, as a result, some pets become rather special to me as I treat them for their illnesses.

This means that sometimes a pet which I am treating becomes a little extra-special. Perhaps as a result of great bravery or simply because that pet copes with all the pain and distress of a grave illness with enormous courage and fortitude!

Toby Ellis is one such dog, to whom I became very close during his ordeal this week. He is a twelve year old black and tan cross labrador, with a look of gentleness and tranquillity which melts you from the inside out. Perhaps he shows the same qualities as his mum, who bravely supported the major surgery that he underwent during Tuesday morning.

He was reported as 'slowing down' over a two to three week period, and certainly seemed under the weather.

We x-rayed his abdomen, and there we saw the offending mass, located somewhere behind the liver. Now came the hard decision! Should we operate or not?

With his owner's permission we decided to find out what was going on, and proceeded to perform a laparotomy operation, which allows visualisation of the organs inside.

My worst fears were confirmed! It was a tumour, the size of a grapefruit, attached to the caudal lobe of the liver. The only answer: to remove the growth. An infrequently performed procedure, and fraught with danger of blood loss and complications in the blood-vascular system.

We decided to go for the dangerous option, and remove the mass. But within seconds a massive bleed began due to the tumour rupturing when handled.

Everyone swung into action. A transfusion began, and as I struggled with the operation, my nurses fought to keep all vital signs under control. All of us were consumed by the need to succeed!

Two hours later the weary team placed the last suture, and Toby was taken into intensive care, where for the next eighteen hours he received round the clock attention from the nurses, willing him to survive.

In the words of dear old Rolf Harris, it genuinely was 'Touch and go' for those first few hours, and brave Toby remained very weak, but stable for the whole night.

Mrs Ellis rang regularly every couple of hours, and the news remained grave. I remained unsure of whether the 'old boy' would pull through, but I left him to the night care of one of my colleagues.

It was my day off the next day, but I couldn't keep away, and with a heavy heart, I slipped into the practice just after eight in the morning.

It is a long walk from the reception into the kennels, and I fully expected to see an empty kennel, where Toby had been recovering the previous evening It was! But next door, in the middle of the biggest 'tailwag' that you could imagine was Toby, looking as if nothing very important had occurred. He clearly felt in need of breakfast and getting home!

What a hug I gave him! Our teamwork had done the job, but I gave him all the credit, and he proved me correct because his recovery so far has been remarkable, with no complications... What a dog!

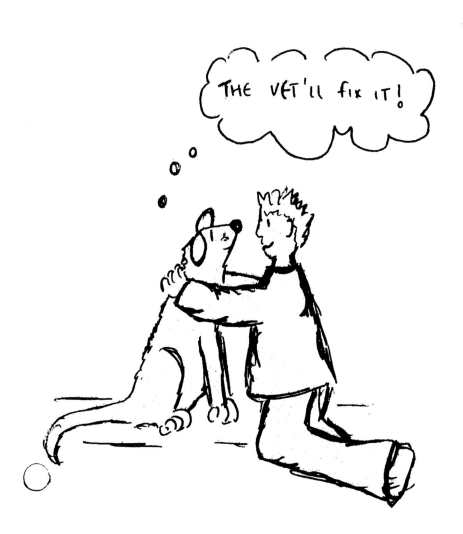

Special Christmas advice

I have always supported the need to prevent unwanted pets ending up in the Christmas stocking, but have you ever considered how Santa manages to get those small pups and kittens down the chimney!

In all seriousness, I have frequently needed to advise clients on the behaviour of their new pets over the Christmas period, rather than dealing with them being 'unwanted'.

A caller on Christmas day once asked me to help the budgie that had been bought for his mother. He reported that it had sadly fallen from its perch into the gin bottle and was now singing out of tune!

He managed to hold out during the ten seconds silence that I afforded him, before obviously collapsing at the other end of the phone in guffaws of laughter.

The following year, while on call again over the festive period, I was 'dogged' by regular calls from a lovely lady who had received a bouncing baby great dane on Christmas morning.

Her first call to me was at 7.30 am, to report that he had eaten six mince pies, and his stomach was swelling - but he was bright and well, and resting.

I advised her to keep the pup quiet, perhaps on his own, well away from any possible 'edibles', and to ring me in an hour, should his stomach continue to swell.

Two hours later, the same lady rang again. 'I locked him in the sitting room while we all had breakfast,' she began. 'Then I heard a bang. We all rushed through and he'd chewed through the electrics for the Christmas tree.'

'How is he?' I asked.

'Well, he looked a bit surprised, and all his hair is singed round his mouth.'

'He wasn't knocked out then?...'

My words trailed off as she began to scream at someone, or something in the background, 'Stop it... now!... get him off there! Oooooo!'

It took about a minute to restore normal service. The lady returned to the phone 'It's alright, he was pulling at the Christmas tree. He seems to be a bit of a handful.'

'Hmmmmm,' I agreed. 'How's his stomach?'

'Yes, alright, but I want to know what to do with him?'

'Well, he obviously is becoming so excited that his exuberance overwhelms the situation! Try to keep him as quiet as possible, but pay him regular attention. Try to make him feel part of the family but stop him becoming too excited.'

Looking back, I said nothing of any real substance, so as I sat down to my Christmas lunch, I should not have been surprised to get another call from the worried puppy owner.

'He's swallowed a bag of chocolate money!' she half yelled down the phone.

'All of it ?'

'Yes! I managed to grab the net bag from his mouth, but he's got the lot, including the bits of metal foil they were wrapped in.'

I decided that she should continue to monitor him for the next hour, and ring if he was sick or seemed uncomfortable. It was likely that he would pass the lot from the other end.

Instead, I rang her, needing to satisfy myself that the litle fellow was Ok.

At last he was asleep, comfortably. 'He's such a super little chap,' she reported.

There is a moral to this story!... Your pup can seriously damage your Christmas day, and may seriously interfere with your vet's Christmas lunch.

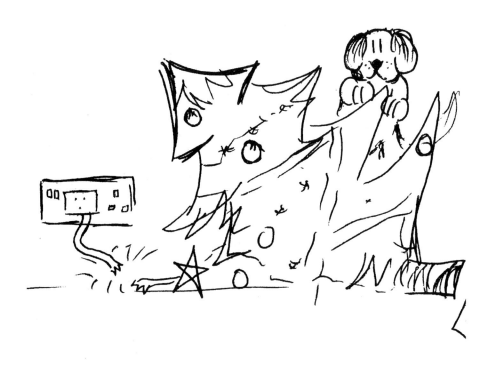

Timmy and Hobnob's opinion on seeing things clearly

There are few things we humans value more than our ability to see clearly, enabling us wonder at life and everything!

I was minded of this last week, while reading an article in our local weekend magazine about the advances in cataract surgery in human medicine, where Norwich is considered a centre of excellence.

In less than fifteen years, progress has been made from rather unpleasant surgery, usually requiring special glasses afterwards to facilitate vision, to present day microsurgery, enabling removal of the offending lens and replacement with a foldable plastic prosthesis through a tiny, self healing wound; during a procedure which can take only fifteen minutes, conducted under local anaesthetic.

There are similar centres of veterinary excellence, for example, at Newmarket, where a comparable pet operation is available. But the catch is that it has to be performed under general anaesthetic, and it can cost upwards of a thousand pounds!

Cataracts are one of the most misunderstood ocular diseases in human and veterinary medicine! Most folks have a concept of some sort of skin growing over the eye: but it is no such thing, being simply an increase in opacity and density of the lens, preventing light passing through successfully.

The wonderful new technology-enabling microsurgery is hugely expensive (the machines alone can cost eighty thousand pounds) hence, when I was removing cataracts from a couple of my patients' eyes recently, I had to resort to the more surgically intensive methods. Don't get me wrong! This operation still works very well, and can transform a dysfunctional pet, giving it a new lease of life.

Timmy, a small, determined little yorkie, who always appeared to rather like me, was the first to have his sight partially restored. After a long operation, and several weeks of eye drops, he greeted me, wagging his tail. I was delighted! I reached down to give him a coax, and he promptly tried to bite me. Years of blindness had not blunted his ability to remember the correct person to chomp when, at last, he could actually see him.

My second patient, Hobnob, is a steadfast, long-haired chihuahua. His owner reported him following her, and pin-pointing biscuits for the first time in ages, at his post-op check. Yet, when I carried out all my tests to prove that he could see, he simply stared straight ahead, pretending nothing had changed, until I caught him out, with a deftly-flicked piece of cotton wool, 'googlied' across his field of new vision. He threw a cursory glance at it, then continued eyeballing the distance.

I briefly thought about the wonder and gratitude that must be felt by human patients when successful sight restoration occurs. I presume that Timmy and Hobnob had presupposed that they had seen the last of me for several years as their respective sights waned. What a shock to to realize that the same 'old duffer' still existed. It deserved a nip and a cold shoulder.

29

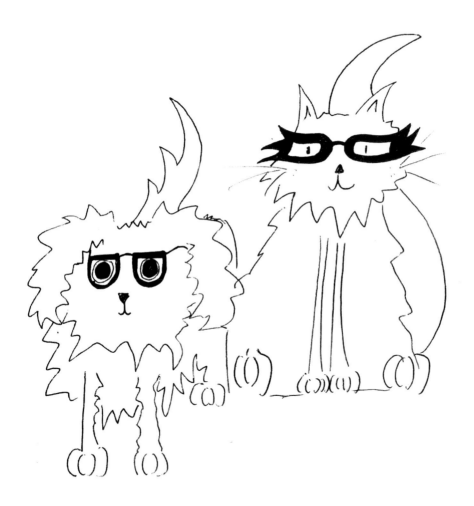

A new home for an unwanted dog

When a dog is a much-loved member of the household, affectionate and devoted to its owners, it is easy to fall into the habit of assuming that he or she thinks like a human being… It said that in a book that I read on dog psychology.

But how do you think a dog feels when that same family sees that dog as a burden or frustration? And looks to re-homing or abandonment.

Thankfully, that same dog doesn't have the same complex cognitive processes of we humans, and has no ability to brood over the past, worry about the future, or most importantly, think in any way symbolically.

Does this mean that the little dog left with us at the clinic last week because the owners were splitting up, had no concern about its dilemma? I think not. She was very concerned to eat as much as possible and attach herself to every member of staff, and socialise with my dogs, and any other that would extend the hand of friendship!

She became 'the practice dog' and showed herself off to numerous clients, wagging her tail and rolling onto her back to order with such frequency that she was also named, 'The Seal'. Vicky, one of our nurses was her favourite, and she followed her endlessly around the clinic, giving advice on any subject that came to hand.

She was, and still is, a charming little dog. But just as the practice policy that any healthy, fit, but unwanted pet is signed over to us for re-homing is enforced, the policy that those pets must go to new homes, and not prove an extra burden to the charities is also adhered to.

Sadly, our little dog was taken away by its new owner this week. It was a moving parting, with all of us saying goodbye and giving her a farewell cuddle. Not that she was concerned. Her new home is ten acres of farm and stables set in deepest Norfolk, with a new mum and dad who have years of experience with her breed.

Tonight, I had a phone-call from the new owner. She reported that her new charge was as delightful as promised. Her love of food, companionship and following humans was undiminished, but she had found a few 'new tricks', including ingestion of copious amounts of horse dung and serial attacks upon the waste bin, where the only evidence of the culprit was a short, stumpy tail, wagging furiously from within the bin itself, and a trail of refuse spread across the kitchen floor.

In fact, her ability to eat has landed her with a new name… 'Dyson' The only vacuum without the need to change the bag!

So, another happy ending, and proof that our pet dogs can adapt well to frequent change of owner and environment; but yet again, even more proof that we humans cannot help but treat our pets as 'little humans'. This story is a point in fact. We all spent all week at the clinic doing that very thing, and it's much more fun than all that psychoanalysis.

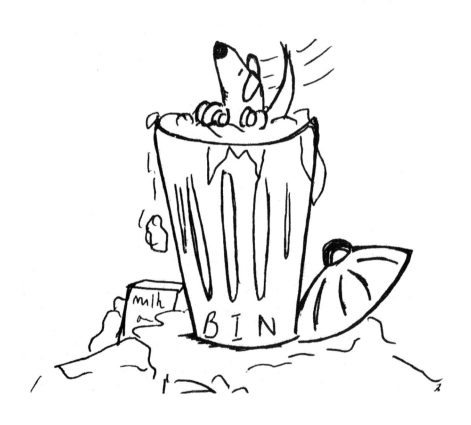

Teddy's thoughts on the plaster on his broken leg

I got taken into the 'bad place' today! When I'd finished play-fighting with Humphrey next door, he chased me out of his drive and into the road, where everything suddenly went blank!

When I came round, my left leg really hurt, and when I looked at it, it bent the wrong way! I tried to stand up, but it just gave way, and did it hurt!....There were lots of the upright animals standing round me at the side of the road. That was scarey, so I hissed a lot and gave them one of my angry looks. They wouldn't go away. I wanted to get somewhere to hide and lick this leg.

One of them picked me up, which wasn't too bad, but he smelt of the 'bad place'! He laid me on a soft thing that had the smell of the 'four legs' (you know, the barking things that chase us if we go in their gardens) and held my neck quite tight as he pushed something sharp and painful into it. I yowled a bit, but very quickly became all 'woozy'. I couldn't hold my head up and it all went dark again.

Next thing, I woke up with a white box surrounding me, and bars in front. I vaguely remembered this from when I was six months old. Something happened which stopped me getting so angry, and I didn't want to spray up the curtains anymore. I don't know exactly what happened, but that wasn't very nice either!

Upright animals were staring into the white box, making noises. I could smell other smells of the 'bad place' where my owner takes me in that dreadful basket a couple of times each year: when the person in the green tunic usually sticks something sharp into my neck! And then rams a white thing into my mouth to make me froth, which he says kills worms. It's funny because when my owner tries to do it, I can always spit it back at him.

I realised that my leg didn't work, but at least it seemed to point the right way round, even though it dragged behind, and had sticking stuff all round it. Every time I tried to move, it wouldn't follow like usual, so I got really angry and tried to yowl at it, but it still wouldn't come in the right direction.

Eventually, I laid down and just stared at it. I didn't understand!

An upright she-animal kept leaning into this white container and coaxing me and trying to offer me bits of food, and sometimes stuck something sharp into my neck or bottom. Then she wrote something on the front of the papers on the cage.

It was a very strange place! At night I cried out a little bit in case someone would come in to let me out. The solid lump round my leg was so annoying.

It doesn't hurt so much now. It's been four days and nights, and believe it or not, the uprights who live in my house came to see me today, letting me put some of my smell on them at last. It was nice to smell me and my territory again, and to find someone worth putting some of my odour on. It reminded me that I can't wait to get back and sort out that Humphrey again.

I overheard one of the uprights talking about me going home tomorrow. I can't wait, because now I can support myself on that lump where my leg used to be. Perhaps I will be able to get the lump off if I keep licking and chewing at it. Then I can climb a tree, and go upstairs and hide under one of the beds or even get out into the garden to do a bit of sorting out! Thank goodness I didn't make it too easy for them, though I suspect that they'll get me back inside the 'bad place' at some point in the future!

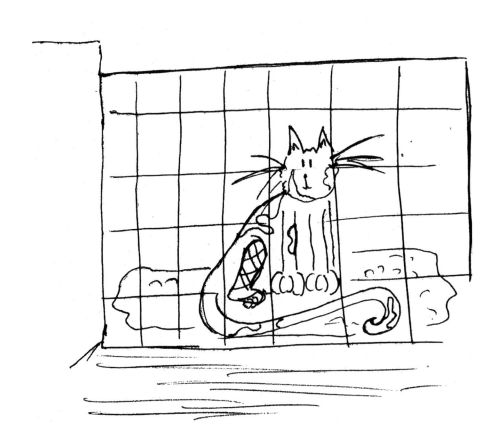

The Trick is in the Click

I love new toys, particularly those that are simple and provide maximum fun and entertainment, so when I received a free sample of a new toy at the practice, I had to be the first to try it out. Unfortunately, I hadn't realised that this new invention would have limitations!

Well it's not really a new invention, more a simple device described as the 'training revolution for dogs', based upon a theory called 'operant conditioning', which is a relatively new way of training your dog, where you teach it to respond regularly to something that positively reinforces and stimulates the appropriate action!

Are you with me so far? I hope so, because you will be underwhelmed by this new toy called 'The Clicker', which is a small, finger-operated device, giving a sharp, metallic, snapping noise when pressed; which can be used as a conditioned reinforcer. In plain terms, the dog hears the click, which he or she learns is always followed by something nice, like a sweetie, and so the action is repeated to gain the reward, but is initiated by the clicking noise. It's a sort of training tool - and I'm sure it has a valuable place in training.

But nobody had told our three year old dog, Wellington. He's really nice, but slightly deficient in the old grey cells - hence my desire to try my new toy on him specifically, in an attempt to prove it can work. You see 'Welly' has an annoying habit of releasing high decibel noises, a cross between a yelp and a bark at any time, without any apparent reason or cause.

I read the instructions carefully 1) Click, then treat 2) Click while the behaviour is happening 3) The click marks the end of the behaviour, so let the dog stop and eat the treat 4) Only click once! Etc.etc.etc.!

Wellington barked, and continued to bark at nothing at six-thirty in the morning, while on his regular walk down the lane. I fumbled in my pocket, grabbed the Clicker and pressed it hard, close to his left ear, while holding a small piece of biscuit as a reward for the expected response.

He stopped alright, reacting to the noise, but saw the biscuit, grabbed it from my hand and dashed headlong into the distance, making a strangled, gurgling-type of noise, as he tried to eat the biscuit while on the run and bark at the same time... What a success! Stuff the dogs, I thought, let's try this technique on a totally new breed.

I advanced purposefully toward Jelly Bean, our new kitten, who certainly needs to know her place. She's far too well-socialised, and at eight weeks old, needs a firm hand.

I showed her the Clicker... She prepared to pounce. I clicked! She pounced, sinking her 26 baby teeth and 18 claws simultaneously into my left hand. I dropped my Clicker onto the parquet floor, where it was rapidly pounced upon by small cat, who proceeded to kick it around the floor for five minutes, having a great game.

Clickers retail for several pounds via the internet and several reputable pet magazines, but where do I advertise them second hand? Or can I trade it in for one of those Stress Shooters? They are brilliant!

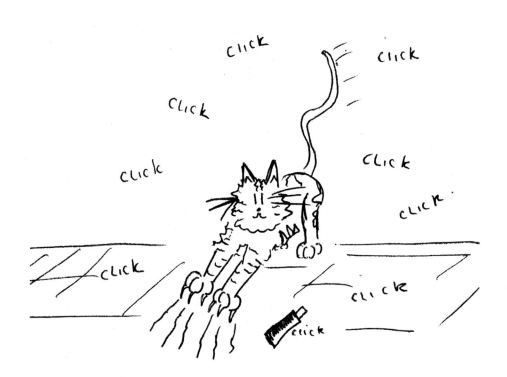

Phoebe - the bionic cat

If I had to choose one species that I treat for an ability to recover from the most dramatic injuries, then it would be the cat.

There are many colloquial comments that perfuse the veterinary profession which relate to the historical powers of repair amongst other fine qualities of the domestic feline, particularly, as an example, relating to the mending of shattered bones caused by road traffic accidents.

One old sage of the profession once told me not to worry about a broken femur mending because, 'All you have to do is show one broken end to the other and it will mend.' Another regularly stated,'It's a cat, it'll be alright.' Essentially referring to the regularity with which apparently hopeless cases of bone damage healed without complication.

One such case of mine i.e. apparently hopeless, was a delightful little female cat called Phoebe, brought in some weeks ago by a caring Samaritan who, as so often happens, found her injured and just about alive, lying by the side of the road.

She was in a sorry state. Bleeding from a damaged jaw, with a pelvis and two back legs which rattled like a bag of loose bones. In fact her left hindleg hung limply, where all the muscles of her thigh had been torn away.

I wrestled with my conscience as to whether we should even try to help in any other way than releasing her from her pain and misery. We had the added problem of no owner to consult.

But, in the middle of examining her, she popped her head into my hand and started purring, not with fear, but with, 'I mean you no harm' at being coaxed. She was a cat! She would be fine.

The following day I set about putting everything back in relatively the right place. Her right femur was so badly shattered that it needed a pin and three retaining wires to hold all the fragments of bone together, while her left hip was so squashed that the hip joint no longer existed, and the head of the femur was dislocated two inches from where it should have been.

Her left pelvis was broken in three places, requiring screws and wires to haul the pieces back into position. There! It was all done. Time to sit back and see if Phoebe could function.

She could! The next day she was taking weight on her left leg. I winced as she attempted to use her litter tray, but she made it, and within three days seemed to be rapidly recovering and free from severe pain.

I've seen her regularly with her new owner in the last few weeks and the recovery is going swimmingly. Via our colleagues at the RSPCA, yet again, she has been looked after and delivered to a brand new owner. She hobbles a little bit on her right leg, but is now trying to jump up if given the opportunity. She is a marvel and testament to that statement,'She'll be alright! She's a cat!'

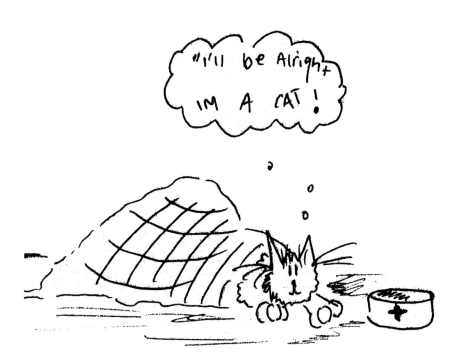

Puppies on all sides

So there I was! Yet again telling Chester that he should prepare a special cage for the long recovery period required for a badly injured road traffic accident cat which I had repaired on Monday afternoon (yet another remarkable story of a cat's ability to survive horrific injuries and bounce through surgery as if that was all that was needed), when he interrupted me to whisper, "Come over here… move quietly".

I was at one of the RSPCA kennel facilities, where so many of the unwanted, unloved, un-owned animals are offered sanctuary, and the chance of a new beginning. Chester, the best dog handler I have ever known, and kennel owner, was about to show me fourteen of his most demanding charges.

Sitting in two adjacent kennels were the two groups of seven. They had to be split up because they were just too much all together - too much of everything from both ends!

There they all sat, scrunched up on each of the single, raised bed, looking too big for those beds, which had provided warmth and comfort for several weeks, wriggling with delight, as someone looked as if they might pay them some attention; tails winding up the excitement, until they could hold on no longer. They began to climb all over each other, tumbling headlong to greet us. Heads were squashed and tails chewed on the way.

This motley crew of fourteen pups were born at the kennels to a gentle lurcher called Rosie, nine weeks ago. Her sweet nature has remained undaunted during the nine weeks of being eaten out of house and home. She still seems to smile whenever you give her a cuddle, and never fails to match up to her responsibilities. It has amazed me that a pregnant bitch, dumped unceremoniously upon the RSPCA, has still maintained such a soft and friendly attitude toward humans.

Those rascal pups have acquired most of her good points, and a few, no doubt, from their unknown father, who, I presume, might have been a boxer or boxer-cross, because all the pups have a tinge of boxer look about their faces, yet retain mum's brindle and white shaped body.

They have had regular check-ups from all the vets at the clinic, but I remember fondly giving them an MOT prior to splitting up the group, at around six weeks of age. What was so funny was the way in which each pup, while being given the once over, dangled limply in our arms, with mouths wide open, gently shaking with the stress of it all. They neither resisted nor complained until it was over, resuming chomping upon any closely available appendage belonging to the nearest sibling.

Only one sticks out as the 'gang' leader. He was always the biggest, from rugrat to fully functioning puppy; always in trouble, but prepared to take the consequences. I will leave those of you who know us at the clinic to fathom why we nicknamed him 'Rosser'

If only I had taken my camera with me, to capture that perfect picture of all those pups, turning as one to see what was up, as Chester and I crept in!

P.S. All pups, with full MOT, still available. Enquire at your nearest RSPCA office, Norwich. By the way, don't go into their kennels. It's like having a bath in live puppies!

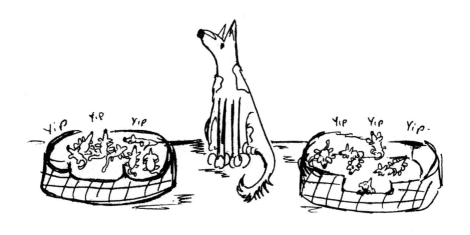

For the dogs with or without a head for heights

As you may be aware, I take great pleasure and regular amusement from what people say about their pets, and from the things that those pets do.

Take, for example, the comments of a client who, this week, had brought his bitch in for a 'morning after' contraceptive injection. Well it was three days after the event, but who's counting!

A second injection is required to ensure that the pregnancy is successfully prevented; and after this, the owner gently reported that he didn't blame her for it happening. I presumed that he meant the neighbour, whose dog had waltzed over an eight foot fence for his 'carnal' experience - but no! He meant that he didn't blame the bitch for allowing the dog to mate with her!

I nodded an assurance that belied my confusion because I really didn't want to enter a discussion about promiscuity amongst our four-legged friends.

But that conversation made me think about the things that our pets get up to and the way in which we so frequently misinterpret or misrepresent those actions. I think that I can advise every pet owner on rationalising the behaviour of their pets... Don't try!

A year old labrador, called Trickster, who is a 'canny' lad at the best of times, visited the clinic for his annual vaccination today. His owners were still stunned and amazed by an incident this week.

He jumped up to greet a member of the family, while in her bedroom, upstairs, then proceeded to bounce onto a table under the window and straight through the upstairs window into the void below!

The screams of terror and the rush of family members into the garden, where they expected to find a badly injured dog, were unfounded, because there was Trickster, wagging his tail - none the worse for his experience and delighted with the attention this episode had provided. He had landed on the soft grass below, and no doubt would have no hesitation in doing the same thing again!

We laughed about his madness, and yet again, I couldn't give the owner one rational reason for his behaviour: rather like the owner who had a lovely little collie-cross, who suddenly became frightened of anything in the air, after some hot air balloons gently glided over her garden. For several months this little dog was a prisoner at home because of the fear of anything up in the sky!

Eventually, I had to dispense a course of 'Doggy Prozac' for a month to defuse this irrational phobia. This worked, and now the fear has totally vanished.

I can't tell you exactly why this dog so suddenly became obsessively fretful, or how the use of an anti-anxiety drug worked so successfully, and apparently reversed the symptoms permanently, but, this is the point of this article - sometimes it is too complex to try.

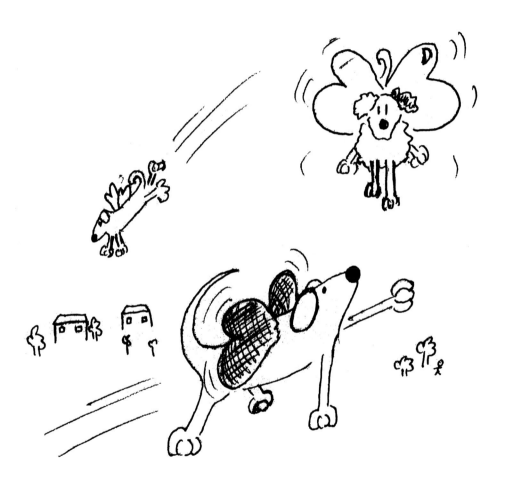

A Slice of American Pie

We've just returned from our holidays, and in keeping with such an event in the Roe household itinerary, I would like, as ever, to share some of the events and meetings with animals and their owners from foreign lands.

This holiday was a bit special, because we travelled to Vancouver, then San Francisco, and eventually to Arizona, to view the Grand Canyon, and animals appeared regularly along the way.

Initially, I thought that nobody owned a pet in Vancouver, but slowly the odd dog-walker appeared, usually with a lovely scruffy mongrel in tow. There seemed to be very few pedigrees, and no cats at all. I didn't see one veterinary practice and no pet shops. Oh dear! I thought. Nothing to write about when I get home!

But San Francisco saved me! It is a city full of quirky owners and their pets. On Fisherman's Wharf we found a street-trader, plying his wares with a little poodle sat up on a shelf, wearing a full doggy morning suit and a pair of glasses, gently sunning itself and fluttering his little eyelashes at all who passed by. He seemed totally happy; as was the maine coon cat which we met walking round a small shop in Sausolito (just up the coast). The shop, called 'Tails by the Bay' is dedicated totally to selling dog and cat utensils, art and personal presents of unique character. The cat owner kept his cat on a lead and walked everywhere with it, and told us that a visit to this shop was a real treat for it.

As we walked close to Union Square the following day, I nearly gave my wife more kittens, as I yelped with glee at the sight that I beheld. For walking out of a shop were two Chinese ladies with their little lhasa dogs, each with individually dyed ears and tails - believe me! One had pink ears and tail, while the other had matching green. I was in heaven, accosting the poor owners, demanding a photograph, which I will share with all on request, when it's developed.

At last, I thought! This holiday was throwing up just what I needed. But all was topped by the battered Nissan car I caught sight of as we left the city to drive to Arizona.

I released more than a squawk of laughter this time, because the driver had something unusual as his passenger, which sat on the back of the car passenger seat. As the driver turned left or right, both he and the passenger leaned to the left or right. It was hilarious!

His passenger was a parrot! But sadly the video camera could not be torn from its case before car, driver and parrot leaned their way off into a side street.

We left San Francisco, heading east, where the heat and dryness means fewer people and more specialised wildlife. We all froze when we overheard a shop owner whispering too a friend, asking whether the rattlesnake that he had bashed with a stick the previous day and thrown into a flowerbed nearby, had shown itself! But this was all forgotten when, the following day, we all sat watching the sun set over the Grand Canyon at Yavapai point. One of nature's finest sights! Unfortunately, we almost missed it, because right below our feet, two little chipmunks were gathering supper, twitching and jinking around, on the edge of a vertical, five thousand foot drop! These little things nearly stole the show.

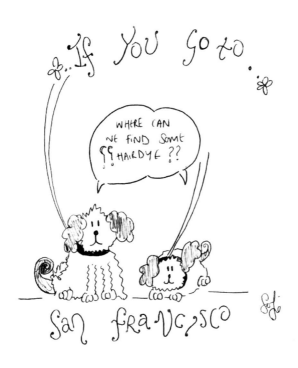

Blimey, another tortoise!

It is that time of year again! You may be happily watching the premature buds bursting for life, or the activity of the song birds, collecting bits and pieces for those early nests, but, spare a thought for the pet tortoise, whose life has been turned upside down by the mild climate pervading our shores over the past few years.

Now in the good old days, when John Noakes could happily show us how to put your tortoise into cardboard box, full of straw, ready for a decent sleep up in the attic, and give a totally believable 'Blue Peter' promise that nothing would stir until the early in the following spring, Britain had a reasonable freeze during the winter. Not so now!

Our humble, much-loved little chelonians suffer premature wake up syndrome with ever-increasing frequency these days; and I have to deal with their inappetance, weight loss and dehydrated state as best I can.

This week, Peanuts, among others, arrived as usual, for an early check up after a pretty poor hibernation, which was quite worrying because he had woken up too early in the previous year, requiring hospitalisation for nearly two weeks and careful stomach tubing to get him into a reasonable state, to begin eating on his own and to store enough body fat, making him fit for the next 'big sleep'.

Suffice it to say that Peanuts did not gain enough weight, so we had advised against allowing him to hibernate last autumn - but he had other ideas, escaping into the garden one day, eluding capture and making for the compost patch, where a decent snooze began.

So here he was! Underweight, but active, and attempting to outrun me before I could put him on the scales to assess him. A multivitamin injection and advice on giving him a week to start eating before we intervened again, sent him on his way. In a way, I won't mind if he returns for a stay, because he has a marvellous, sociable habit of pushing the vivarium glass door open and popping an inquisitive head out for a regular chat.

Then Tony arrived: a tortoise that had not eaten for a month since his premature alarm call. He is still with us, undergoing intensive feeding, a specialist stimulatory lighting regime and treatment with fluids to correct salt and water imbalances.

I didn't presume any more could arrive! But Sophie and Henry arrived on the very same day, thankfully fit and well, but requiring insertion of an identichip tagging device, which goes under the loose skin of the right hindleg, where I also insert a small suture afterwards to prevent the microchip popping out. I also hospitalise for a few hours afterwards, to make sure there is no bleeding to be concerned with.

All went well until I was informed that Sophie, the smaller of the two, had decided to play a game called 'Eat Henry's head', which involved snapping at Henry's nose, then chasing him round the cage as he made his getaway!… such goings on! Tortoises ain't what they used to be!

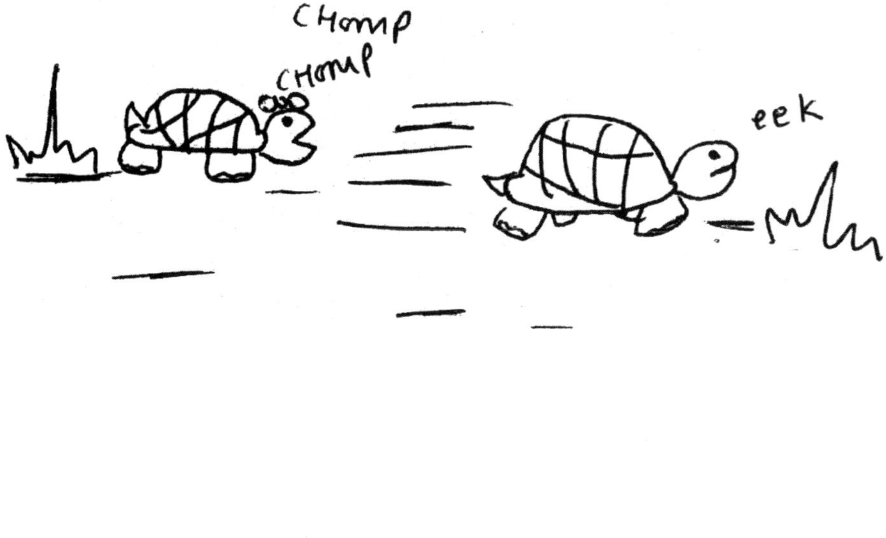
CHOMP
CHOMP
eek

Bluebell makes a run for it

For so many of us, the enjoyment of a holiday, such as Christmas or the New Year can be spoilt by the need to be separated from much-loved pets. So it seems that lots of clients nowadays take their pets with them on trips to friends or family.

Bluebell, a little female cat and her brother, had to go with mum and dad to Brighton for the festivities, where her usual escape pranks, regularly witnessed and frequently curtailed by vigilant folk at RAF Coltishall (where she lives), would not be tolerated.

It would be reasonable to presume that concern for Bluebell would not be required while in Brighton, staying away from home – strange environment and all that. But she had further ideas!

The owner received a call on his mobile just after nine on a morning following Christmas, from someone thirty miles away from Brighton.

'Errr.....Hello, I've got your cat with me at work! I'm in Staines!'

'What!' the owner squirmed.

'I've got your cat. I phoned the number on her collar. You are the owner of a cat called Bluebell?'

The caller went on, 'I was taking my dogs for a walk at about six-thirty this morning, and met your cat, walking alone through the park. She seemed quite at home, wandering around, but when she came over for a chat, I thought I'd better check her out. That was when I found your mobile number on her collar.'

Bluebell could not have been much luckier. The Samaritan had taken her to work, thinking that it was far too early to ring the number he had found – what a great guy!

So the owner slept on, blissfully.

How these events had unfolded was quite remarkable, in as much as she obviously had an accomplice helping with her escapade and duplicity. In fact, it's her kid brother cat, who has the knack of being able to open doors!

He had apparently released the latch on the outside door of the lobby in which the cats were staying during Christmas, enabling Bluebell to wander off. Yet he stayed put, as ever, too scared of trouble or convinced that he had done his job. Or perhaps he thinks she'll really cop for it this time.

This seems to be a game, enacted frequently by the two of them, allowing Bluebell to go walk about. But exactly how, and why, she had decided to find a park four miles away to wander to, was a complete mystery!

Did I have a competent and professional answer to prevent this happening again? Yes! Lock all the doors, and thank someone special for the appearance of that Samaritan.

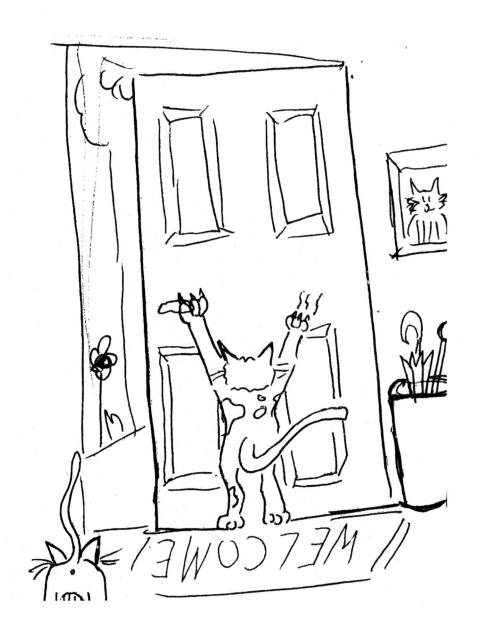

Jelly Bean has come of age

It is now official! Jelly Bean, the tiny kitten, saved from certain death in August, and brought up by family Roe, has become a 'grown up'. Well, not exactly, because she has reached an age where she can be classified as and adult – she is six months old, and feeds on adult food, and is allowed out at all times of the day and night. She can even think about starting a family!

But J.B. Bean is so totally unaware of her new found freedoms and capabilities that I feel she is likely to remain a perennial kitten for all of her life.

She lives a life so remarkably geared towards the relentless extraction of pleasure from her games and antics, pouring abject scorn upon her hapless victims, human and feline, that she could comfortably fill the shoes of Catwoman, the tormentor of Batman.

Her day begins with a well aimed jump onto the bed, landing squarely on the stomach, from where she purrs and chirrups until the human wakes: mission accomplished, she proceeds to sit on your head, curling her little prehensile tail round your face, stomping her small, leather feet in time with her vocalizing.

From there, a game is started involving jumping upon any human extremity sticking out from the bed, sinking teeth and claws simultaneously!

Unless, of course, one of the other cats arrive, in which case she drops us like a stone, preferring to chase them round the upstairs, until they 'pull rank' and sit on her for a few minutes, which usually means she retreats downstairs.

Here we have just found out that she is the culprit who paddles in the pet community drinking bowl. We used to blame poor old Hattie, my little, ageing cavalier, but J.B. has been witnessed sloshing water all over the place, then staring at it as it runs across the kitchen floor.

If admonished for the above, you may consequently find her deliberately pulling lumps of pot-pourri from the bowl on the coffee table, then pretending that they jumped out, all on their own from that pot, so demanding chasing, jumping upon, and even a four-legged pick up and roll into touch!

Her next port of call may be the inside of a lampshade, climbing up the stand and metal framework to reach a point inside, from which she can delicately pat a pretend fly. The lamp usually finishes dejected in a heap of electric cable.

But how can you stay angry for too long? When she can melt your heart by sitting up on her bottom and begging for attention, or by sitting in the catflap, half in, half out, just watching the world go by, suddenly jumping through it, tail all of a swish, running at full pelt into the shrubbery, up into a small tree, then down just as quickly, before sprinting back into the kitchen, via the cat flap. Ending up standing, ready for a fight, hairs all vertical. Then she stops, as quickly as it all began, sits down and licks all four feet lovingly.

She is demonic as often as platonic, and alas, this will all certainly change during the next six months, as maturity spoils the fun, but there's one thing for certain! She's no trouble at all when she's asleep!

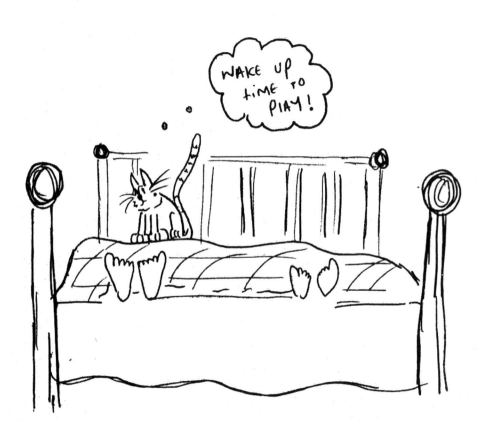

A muddy and wet Wednesday

It was extremely cold on Wednesday morning at 6.30 am. In fact it was wet and extremely cold!

There I was, rummaging through the smelly, wet fronds of some form of all-embracing continental fir tree, looking for a little 'moggie' that a concerned client had found rolling around in apparent discomfort on her front lawn in Felthorpe.

Said moggie was disinclined to be captured, and despite professional blanket throwing, his armoury of rapier-like, clawed legs, and chomping teeth denied us. He was, no doubt, cold, thoroughly disorientated and fearful of our intention.

For a split second I wondered why I did this job! My bed had seemed so appealing when I groaned into action as the emergency bleep woke me up, but I soldiered on, determined that this little fellow was not going to evade me.

Eventually, I made a grab at his tail and dumped him unceremoniously into the cage, rapidly said my goodbyes and drove back to the surgery, wondering exactly what the question (not the answer) was to the quiz on Wally Webb's radio Norfolk early morning show, and why everybody seemed to be getting it wrong!

The next day, this little tom-cat was warm, well fed, and had been named 'Muddy' because of the state in which he arrived. He was purring sociably, eating us out of every type of cat food, and melting everyone's heart, despite his individual 'tom-cat' odour! But still no owner had claimed him.

Yet, as is often the case with cats found in these circumstances, we could not answer why he was showing signs of brain stem disease, leading to totally normal function except inability to use and control the right side of his body. A total mystery existed because there was no sign of a road traffic injury, or other trauma, and all our tests have ruled out infectious diseases.

So Muddy lies in his kennel, soaking up the love and attention. Our colleagues at the RSPCA have agreed to share the costs with us, because no one seems to want him, which has helped us to check for some of the more exotic ailments that might be the cause of his disability.

And that is where you find this bizarre case. Muddy has become a sort of chronic, long-term patient, charming us with his faultless character and manners (after his dodgy start), and I cannot foresee him leaving until he is quite ready. It's one of those situations that I write about so frequently, where an animal's behaviour and demands seems to take over, and we humans look on, helplessly, hooked by the look on that helpless face.

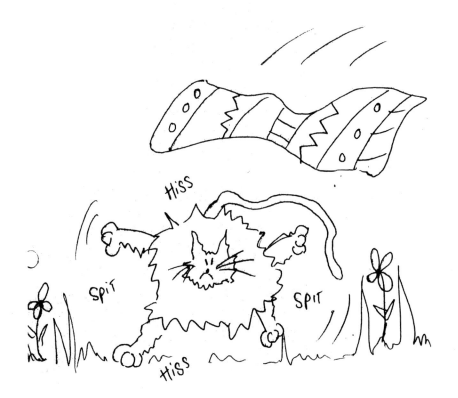

Pet power in New York

It is a well known fact (to the constant annoyance of my family) that whenever I go on holiday, I begin to 'animal-watch'; regularly disappearing to follow somebody or an animal to get a picture or to witness a funny moment of action.

No change then, when on a recent trip to New York, my passion began very early on! You see, to my mind, many New Yorkers regard their pet as something of an accoutrement: a possession, rightly loved and spoilt, but still something to be admired and valued, rather like a monster diamond, dazzling from a digit.

This seed of thought began in Bloomingdales department store, when I espied an obvious, wildly rich woman wandering around with her little lhasa apso in tow; literally being dragged from counter to counter, as she searched for that elusive 'must have'.

My wife and children admonished me as I followed her secretively to get the right camera angle for a picture. I got the impression that madam felt somewhat undressed unless her little dog was with her, rather like the joggers in Central Park. A paradise for me. Who should I photograph first? The joggers with two little chihuahuas, skipping along, wearing identical sun visors to their owners, or the peke, dressed in a 'pukka' burberry raincoat with fur cuff and collar!

It's all part of the rich commune between pet and owner, which I love to observe. But beware, not everybody is a dog lover in Central Park. As we walked down the steps to the fountain, made famous in films like 'Home Alone' and 'One Fine Day' (My wife wouldn't let me pick her up and dance down the stairs, like George Clooney and Michelle Pfeiffer), a menacing character rushed past us speaking into a dictaphone.

As he went past a couple of yapping dachshunds, we heard him report to his tape, 'Man, I hate those dogs!'

Much as the fourteen thousand taxis of New York are vital to transport, the horses and carriages, plying a trade round the park caught my attention.

Our horse, Lady, and her amiable Irish driver, Pat, took us for a delightful night-time trundle. But even Pat managed to break my tranquil relaxation. As I asked him where the horses went at at night (without any knowledge of my profession), he started by complaining about a recent vet's visit to his horse, which cost him, 'a hundret dollars, to test dee blood and heart an' all that!' – bless him. I paid his thirty five dollar fee for a twelve minute stroll without complaint, and determined to keep my identity 'low profile'.

The next day I went back to animal watching, surprised by the number of people who have a mix of three or four completely different breeds of dog in the city, taking them all for regular walks, even along crowded thoroughfares like Fifth avenue.

I asked one owner where the local vet was to be found, and followed directions to Forty sixth street, just off Fifth avenue, expecting a plush, million dollar experience. Instead, I was heartened to find a small building with waiting room directly off the street. Not posh, but warmly decorated with much the same foods on sale as we have at the practice at home; and a small crossbred dog and moggy playing a hearty game of chase in the empty waiting room, unconcerned. It gave me a rather warm feeling of home.

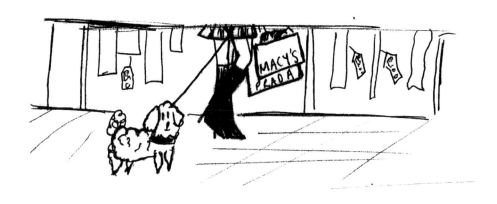

Sasha's futile bid for freedom

I'm very fond of the Rhodesian ridgeback dog: perhaps it's that quirky streak of hairs growing the wrong way all along the back or the idea of a South African dog combining the genes of the bloodhound and the native hottentot species to provide a powerful, majestic breed that oozes energy and athleticism – useful attributes when you were primarily used for hunting big game, especially lions.

Sasha is one such ridgeback whose endurance and hunting skills went a bit awry recently when a thunderstorm scared her so much that she scaled a six foot chain link fence and a screen of trees, to escape from her home in Haveringland.

Admittedly, this storm broke directly overhead and put the fear of the gods into the humans, so goodness knows what she felt like!

Anyway I digress! Sasha went on the run, combing great swathes of distance around Booton, the Witchinghams and Wood Dalling from the Tuesday on which she was lost.

Various Samaritans saw her and reported her presence in these areas but her distraught owners seemed to just miss her as they tore round in her wake. One such sighting even diagnosed her as being a deer on the run!

Tuesday ran into the rest of the week, and the weekend. Adverts were placed everywhere possible and still the stories of the escapee came in thick and fast. She was seen hanging around some horses in a field but ran off when someone got too near: perhaps (her owners thought) she was checking them out because at home she was used to living with equines.

One of the 'just too late' arrivals came when her owners took the other dog, Timmy, with them to try and pick up her scent. They entered an old barn where the obvious excitement of her canine companion suggested that Sasha had holed up there overnight.

As the humans waned, fatigued through nights with no sleep, Sasha followed her instinctive patterns of sweeping across the countryside in huge loops, just like her hunting ancestors, looking for the right scent to enable her to drive any game back to her starting point.

It was all becoming a bit too much by the weekend! Seemingly Sasha would end up getting herself into some trouble soon with a local gamekeeper or passing car and no one could get near her when she was approached.

Then early on Sunday morning a lightly sleeping owner was awoken by unusual noises downstairs – and lo! The little angel had reappeared, albeit tired, hungry and bearing a few scratches and scars for her trouble.

I examined her the following day and pronounced her little the worse for wear, but she nonchalantly offered no word of apology and expressed little remorse for her actions... Well that's children for you!

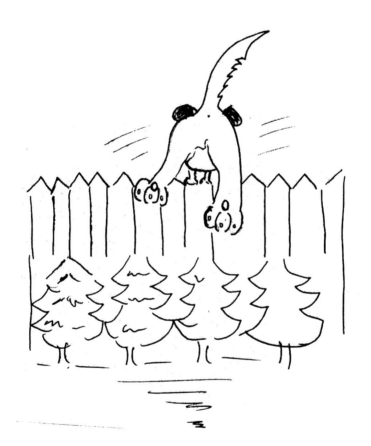

A tight squeeze for an unusual patient

I find it difficult to get up in the mornings; more so when I've been up most of the night already, with a fitting dog, who had settled down nicely by about 3 am.

I was back in bed, just getting comfortable again by four-o-clock, when my bleep burst back into life, 'Please call Norwich police – injured deer.' was all the message said.

I phoned the number. Apparently a deer was stuck in some railings on Colman road, up near the Jenny Lind hospital, which seemed a very strange place for a wild deer to be stuck.

In any event, as I drove round the ring road, marvelling at the large number of people already up and about at such an ungodly hour, I racked my brain for deer doses of tranquillizer, hidden in the depths of a slightly fuzzy, sleep-deprived brain.

It shouldn't have concerned me! I always carry a compendium of drug doses in the car, in the event of coming across an unusual species, or more commonly, forgetting whether such a dose refers to a raccoon or a boa constrictor!

When I arrived, the emergency was a beautiful scene of tranquillity. A tiny female muntjac deer sat in the back of a panda car, wrapped in a fireman's safety bag. Two fire tenders and heavy duty, compressed air pincers had stretched the metal bars like sticks of liquorice, releasing the screaming deer, then squeezed them back together, as if nothing had occurred.

The police and I checked the little deer over for acute injury, but she was fine, just sitting there, as if she believed it to be a 'fair cop' – accepting her fate with aplomb; her shiny, leathery nose twitching, as she stared around, quite relaxed.

We laughed about which direction she was meant to be going in! Had she just finished chomping her way through someone's prize dahlias, in a local garden, and got stuck on the way back, or was she well fed, and in an attempt to return to a tasty feeding area, chosen the wrong gap in the railings, that was just shy of her weightwatchers limit?

Whether she was indeed coming or going was immaterial. As she sat confidently on my passenger seat, I felt as if I had a companion with me! We chatted about this and that on the way back – me doing most of the talking, of course. Her demeanour was quite amazing for a wild deer: she was so relaxed, which is very unusual. I would have expected screams of fear, struggling and much stress, but she appeared to be taking everything in, with great interest!

Back at base, I checked her again: dressed some minor grazes on both flanks; gave her some pain relief for a slightly sore back leg; made her a bed of straw, and finally left her to rest, clambering back into the car, hoping to grab a last hour or so of sleep myself.

Most clients deserve my apology for the following day, when my lack of sleep resulted in some extremely funny malapropisms and general inability to communicate accurately. As for our little Muntjac! She took another lovely ride up to the RSPCA wildlife hospital. Just another 'away day' for her, I suppose.

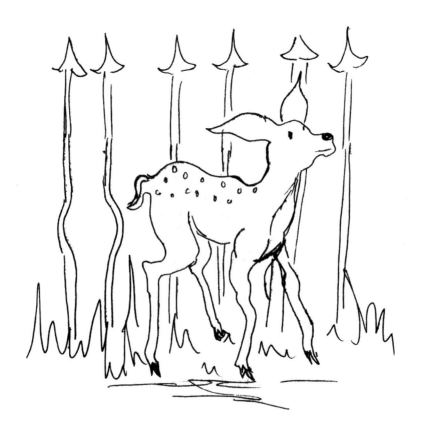

A little extra help at the clinic

His hair is grey with a smattering of white. He wears a stiff collar and weighs in at a round five kilos. He is the latest member of the team at the clinic and he has superb social skills, and though unsure of his alphabet, gives of his best at the computer.

I refer not to hired help, but to a small cat called Cody, who captured the heart of every member of the practice during a longer than acceptable stay with us, while we tried to heal a nasty, chronic skin lesion on his face, which he scratched endlessly whenever his elizabethan collar was removed, undoing three weeks of healing in five minutes!

Sadly, his original owners, who had taken him on after a long stay with the RSPCA (during which time the skin lesion developed), were unable to look after him due to circumstances beyond their control. So in short, when everybody asked for my opinion, I decided to make him 'the practice cat'. Next job is to have a little 'practice cat' lapel badge made up.

Strong words, drug regimes and several experts input had got us nowhere in healing his itchy wound. So as soon as he became 'ours' the collar went on twenty four – seven, and the process of training Cody to become attuned to wandering all day around the practice began.

Great fun followed, watching him choose his favourite windowsills for birdwatching and sleep. One in particular, is just above a computer (used by my wife) in the office, from where he has managed to switch the printer on, and then delete a days records on her accounting system, with gentle taps from his paws as he hones his I.T. skills.

It is not unusual to be making an appointment on the surgery computer, and while concentrating on the screen, find the whole image change. The culprit? A little grey paw sliding in from the side of the monitor! Just helping, of course. He will even plonk his plastic encased head right on the keyboard in front of you, demanding attention, pressing his face against yours harder than any feline I have ever known.

His protective collar hinders him ever so slightly, making some of his jumps onto cupboards and work surfaces somewhat clumsy. Having missed, he runs for sanctuary to his night-time quarters in a large kennel in the hospital section, from where he will peer for some minutes, before emerging for more mischief.

A character of unfailing warmth, mischief and inquisitiveness, makes Mr. Cody a delightful new member; but he has also taken on duties beyond his remit, involving himself in post-operative care, sitting by kennels containing animals recovering from anaesthesia, staring at the occupant for however long it takes for them to come round.

Sadly while the little man has his collar on, he will not be allowed out and is incarcerated at night. This is the hardest part, because he knows the pattern so well that he has learnt to give us the most plaintive cries as we shut up the surgery for the night, recognising that he's 'banged up' for another twelve hours. I simply remind him of the reasons why he is there, reinforcing that pound for pound, he is the least cost-efficient member of the practice, to which he responds by rubbing up against the bars of his kennel, ignoring my remonstration, fully aware that it might entice me to give him just one final head scratch (or two) before I leave.

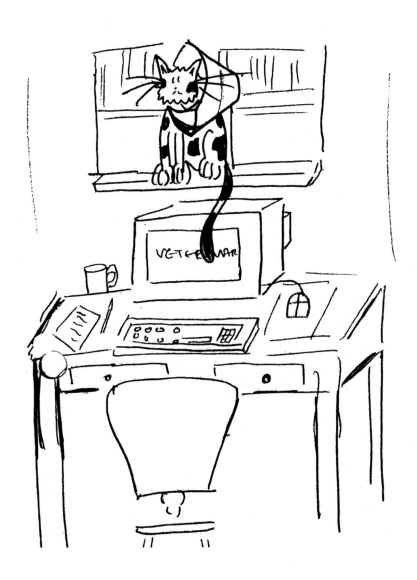

A fond farewell to Mr Cody

It was difficult to believe that he could so nonchalantly accept to fall asleep in the open basket next to a pile of goodies prepared for his imminent departure, but that's Cody (the practice cat for the last six months) for you !

An air of reflection and sadness had pervaded the surgery for most of the day. The little grey and white feline lodger, who had ingratiated himself with us, and who had become a real member of our practice, was off to his new home with one of our nurses, who is expecting her first baby.

'Do you know there's a cat on the loose?' was the most frequent piece of advice given by clients, as he wandered around the clinic, and it was not unusual to see him pop his head from behind the blinds in the waiting room and nearly deliver the 'fear of God' to some unsuspecting client.

Other pets faired just as badly. Cats in baskets were always fair game. He would sit as close as possible, looking inquisitively at the new arrival. The bubble above his head was clearly saying, 'You're in there and, as you can see, I'm out here. Tough luck, eh!'

He was as equally dominant when it came to litter trays, in as much as if you turned your back on an empty cage for two ticks, he'd be in there and make good use of it. We even had to put protective covers over all the 'ready to go' litter trays stacked upon the kennels, because he was not averse to a bit of 'high altitude' penny spending.

Yet sympathy abounded for this little chap, condemned to wearing a protective elizabethan collar to prevent his constant attacks upon an allergic area on the side of his face. Perhaps I should forgive him for his Irish jigs on the computer keyboards or jumping on paper as it spewed from the printers or 'tap-tapping' anything mobile such as pens, syringes, small bottles or their tops right to the edge of any table. When it eventually fell to the floor, he looked at you, then to the object with his wry grin. His face genuinely reflected his state of mind and, in typical human fashion, we concocted the lot! – from grinning to swooning, melting looks as you rubbed his belly, slitty-eyed grimaces when he was being told off! – even his body language told all: head down, walking as fast as possible, usually meant he'd been up to something in the direction from whence he'd come.

The collar prevented him going outside, so he needed vantage points from which to check out freedom: his favourite position was the top of the computer monitor in the prep room, from where he could chatter at the starlings, who whistled their way through early morning courtship. It also allowed him to flick his tail all over the screen, causing increasing annoyance. The more you scolded him, the more he flicked it.

But my abiding memory of Cody was the day after he had spent most of his previous day staring at a particularly large lizard, hospitalised in the vivarium. It had gone home the night before but as soon as he was released from his cage, he went straight back for another look. Whilst finding no lizard there he promptly thought he'd try something new, and pretended to be a large lizard, sleeping blissfully in the reptile house for the rest of the morning.

Cody didn't contribute one penny to his upkeep. He complained bitterly about being 'banged up' each night and he caused endless mayhem, but my goodness! Won't we miss him?

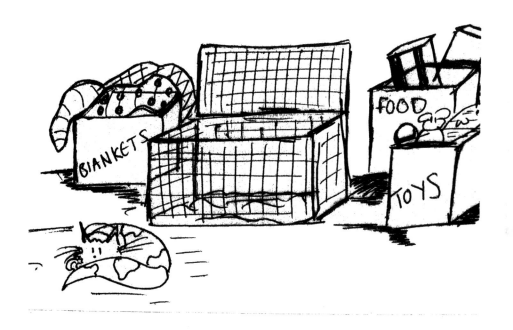

Muddy and Sam
steal the show

There are times when I feel that this column might be turning into a weekly diary, or catalogue of events from the clinic. Yet, in my defence, I most frequently receive comments enquiring about the health of one or more of the pets that I have written about.

So to prevent any sense of loss or causing even one reader to accuse in the fashion, 'I was the last to know', I would like to report that 'Muddy' the wobbly cat from last week is making a remarkable recovery. He can now stand, fully supported on all four legs and, I presume, will return to totally normal function over the coming weeks! Three cheers for 'Muddy. And, by the way, he is not supporting himself solely on his new, rather large, rounded belly!

It is therefore, on the back of such success, that I will tell of the dastardly deed that brought Sam Wilson, an eight month old tabby cat, to the clinic, with a round hole in his right flank. He seemed a little 'off-colour' but not in too much pain - but an x-ray revealed a .22 airgun pellet lodged in his left flank on the opposite side to the hole!

Could the pellet have travelled right through he abdomen of the cat? It had! And an emergency operation revealed six inches of intestine, completely destroyed by this callous shooting incident, which placed the little fellow's life in real danger.

I had to resect the damaged tissue, and surgically join the ends together, hoping that the myriad of possible complications would stay away over the next week of convalescence!

Apart from a few uncomfortable days, Sam healed remarkably well; heading off home with a jubilant mum yesterday. The moment of pleasure taken by some hooligan, in shooting an innocent pet, not only put that animal through pain and suffering, but also reduced his owner to depths of despair that brought a lump to my throat as she tried to cope.

Why do people do these things to helpless animals? I am regularly asked by disbelieving clients. I reply, perhaps with a tinge of cynicism that you've only got to look at what we do to each other to understand the mentality that produces such behaviour!

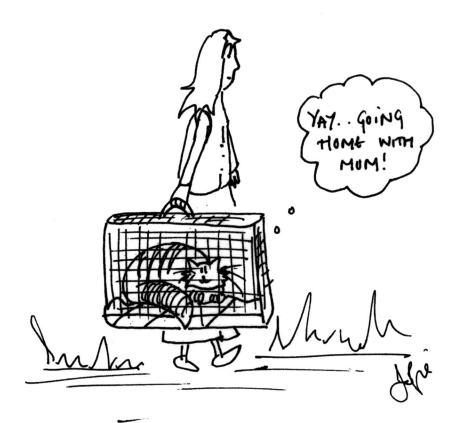

Our pets can read our minds

Don't we just love all those programmes about supposed human powers above and beyond the normal i.e. paranormal. When someone has powers of intuition or extrasensory knowledge, which gives them special faculties?

It is not for me to offer any free service or skill within the practice! But I can offer you a regular inspection of sixth-sense events, without the need for a television licence or a dish-thing. We have our very own 'in house' X-Files.

What is he talking about? I hear you cry! Well, ponder over this! How does Boris, a deaf cat, who visited me today, know when it's breakfast time or when to tumble in for tea? Does that cat have a watch, in-built or otherwise? He surely cannot hear what's going on. So what enables him to be there right on time? His owners assured me that you could set your watch by his timing.

And explain this! Why do so many blind cats function perfectly well within their environment, frequently with owners completely unaware of this. Surely a decent set of sensory whiskers and acute hearing cannot be enough to allow precision movement.

And why do so many cats rather churlishly go missing when an owner is trying to collect them for a visit to the vets? Very frequently they simply are not in the place where they usually would be when the owner goes to find them. I had two sets of clients turn up with only one of a pair of cats for vaccination today, with apologies for the one that had surprisingly gone walkabout.

I joke that they probably hear you making the appointment, or, perhaps more commonly, I suggest, they can read your mind!!!!

Do I really believe this? Well it is certain that our domestic pets really have a brain attuned to the demands of their tough existences from thousands of years ago, which meant survival of only those breeds and types best adapted to take advantage of their environment. In such circumstances, it might be that they have evolved methods of communication which we cannot ever hope to match.

I'm certainly on the case. Aware that we use only a tiny fraction of our brain power, I constantly look for links between human intention and our pets' abilities to pick up the messages.

But, I don't have the faculties to complete my research! Exemplified by my final check of in-patients at the clinic tonight. It was all quiet, as usual. I crept past the kennel in which Vic, the RSPCA cat was sleeping blissfully. He's a delightful chap, but so demanding when awake, that I wanted to leave him snoring. I turned my back to check a drip bag of a cat in the next door kennel, making no sound. Then, as I tried to walk away, my left leg stayed put, pinned by a set of talons!

Vic had grabbed my trouser leg, and pulled it through the cage, realizing that this would demand my attention and, no doubt, a good head and nose scratch.

How did he wake up within seconds and deftly, silently, execute his will, without some special sense that alerted him? (I'm trying to get him to bend spoons next) I've now got a hole in my favourite cords. I need extra faculties. Anyone got any spare?

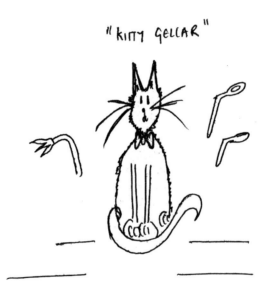

"KITTY GELLAR"

Anyone for fluid therapy?

I have to admit that I was surprised when, last week, I read an article about what was being hailed as the 'Prozac' of the dog world. It suggested that Clomicalm, the drug in question, was akin to the human drug. Not quite, I feel, considering that it is used to reduce anxiety and tension in the dog in the home, and works in a completely different way to Prozac.

The same article also mentioned another veterinary drug, Selgian - again suggesting some form of anti-depressant activity for older dogs, but again, a little bit off-base.

Yet, if such were true, I might have had a little help from such chemicals this week-end, considering the tension and stress, which I suffered as the emergency bleep almost continually summoned me into action, and as I felt like one of those people who keep spinning plates up in the air on sticks.

The reason is that, I had, at one point, four animals on drip-feed fluid therapy in the hospital. It might not sound like much, but I can assure you that when humans are being given intravenous fluids, they stay reasonably still, lying down, accepting the need to preserve the nourishing drip line - just like animals don't!

Cats, in particular, must have read the 'teach yourself' handbook of knots, because they can turn a straight piece of plastic, delivering those fluids into a sculptured work, worthy of Michelangelo, simply by being connected to it.

Dogs, on the other hand, seem to enjoy more varied games, such as 'Exactly how far can you stretch a drip-line before it breaks' or 'If I wrap this round my leg and body, does it make me more likely to get attention'

I knew that I was in for a hard time as I left the hospital for lunch on Saturday, but not quite how! Over the whole weekend I counted up forty seven individual actions, while attending to those drip lines, either flushing, untwisting or re-bandaging etc,etc,etc.

I now suspect that this was all a game; that those pets were deciding which exact form of sabotage to indulge in, while I was away, and consequently taking it in turns.

If you had heard me asking each pet, on all those many occasions 'How did you manage to do that?' you would have perhaps realised more rapidly than myself, that there was 'malice aforethought'. But you see, I genuinely believed those pets to be ill enough that they wouldn't do that to me!

And Oh! By the way, exactly where is the Prozac kept?

P.S For regular readers - Muddy has been rehomed. He is fully recovered. He has officially now left the building!

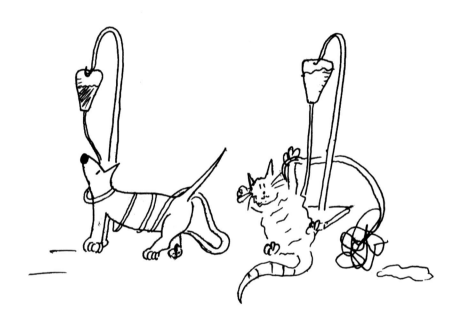

Jelly Bean puts her nine lives to a severe test

Do you operate on your own animals? is a common question put to me in the surgery. 'Only when I have to!' is the frequent reply.

It is really tough carrying out an operation on your own, much loved pets. Imagine a human surgeon doing likewise to a member of his or her family. It sort of goes against the grain.

So my distraught family, bearing a badly damaged Jelly Bean (the little kitten hand-reared by us from a couple of days old) presented a stomach-churning vision.

She has run the gauntlet for several months now, and our natural pessimism over the longevity of an inquisitive cat, who has interests over the other side of the road was being born out.

Thankfully (and I say this advisedly), our small charge was only shown to be suffering from a fractured left tibia and fibula – the bones of the lower leg: but a rather hurried x-ray revealed it to be a rather complicated fragmented fracture of the worst type!

There are so many things to assess before mending a fracture. And Bean's break was rather troublesome. I had to consider the fact that a piece of bone had punctured the skin, increasing the chance of sepsis; that the fracture site was fragmented, and that tibial breaks are very prone to rotate, causing deformity of the lower limb during repair.

I plumped for external fixation, where multiple pins inserted into each part of the bone either side of the fracture are bolted to an adjacent steel bar, which essentially supports the whole framework of the broken bone (having been brought back into the best alignment available with the fragments), while it attempts to heal.

This technique prevents the rotation problem and gives the greatest chance of repair in the face of a potential infection. So there I was, with my little cat anaesthetised in front of me, hoping for my best work.

Two hours later, this little leg was back together. A second x-ray showed good reduction – now it was down to her!

I felt enormous relief; then I began to worry about her post-op care: pain relief, stability of the repair during the six weeks healing; where to keep such a free spirit during that period to prevent complications. All those advisory things that are so easy to tell my clients, but which increase almost out of proportion when it's one of your own.

A pair of dish-like eyes greeted me as she came round from the anaesthetic – her small body no doubt consumed with pain but masked by a generous dose of morphine, to be repeated regularly. During the next few days her pain will decrease, but what worries me is what sort of capers Jelly Bean will get up to in trying to escape her incarceration; what level of complaint we will get from her, and who gets the short straw to have her sleeping in their room at night? Oh yes, teenage daughters do have their uses!

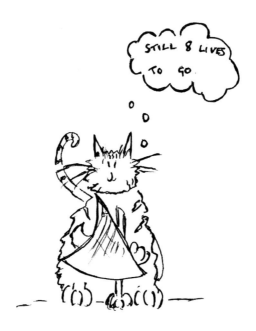

Appreciating Jelly Bean's return to health

Not being loved by every pet that comes through my door comes with the territory. I have convinced myself not too take it personally and have even started a new ruse which craftily covers any potential suggestion of such.

It goes like this! Cat comes into surgery. I take it out of the cage, and cat hisses at me. Owners laugh, and I reply… 'I agree. If I were a cat I'd make it as difficult for the vet as possible.' Thus killing two birds with one stone! In an instant you achieve the shortest possible consultation, ensuring a minimum of treatments and (perhaps more valuably) you prevent the vet from wittering on about all those expensive concoctions for fleas, worms etcetera, hence saving your owner money (vital brownie points here and more cash available for designer sachets of cat food) and making them less likely to shove you in a basket the next time for something that needs tablets etc.

Perhaps a slightly light-hearted approach, but it makes me feel better. And consider this! Today a jack-russell terrier took exception to me examining his foot, turning on me, on a sixpence. Perhaps it was the new glasses accompanying the failing sight, or sheer reflex that speedily removed my hand from the space in mid-air where this little minx chomped a mouthful of nothing?

The crowning glory of the event was the owner's response. He clutched up the little dog and said 'Oh darling! Are you alright?'

Thank goodness for the solace of watching our cat Jelly Bean returning to health from her broken leg. Her pins are causing no problems at the moment, but very early on in her convalescence she caused us all to cringe by taking full weight on her newly-repaired leg and even standing up on just her hindlegs. How animals can cope and seemingly become pain-free after such a terrible ordeal fills me with admiration.

Of greater importance is her mild-mannered approach to incarceration. This feral-foundling, who takes no 'truck' from anybody, has mellowed to a 'chill factor' well below zero. Such things are difficult to explain. I would never be so foolish as to presume any sense of her being beholden to we humans. I just put it down to an early Indian summer. Something has de-tuned her from expressing her more normal feistiness, and I'm going to enjoy it.

You may hear a different story after a further four weeks - the time she still needs to approach full repair. I cannot imagine her patience lasting too much longer. In a way, I hope when she comes back home she will re-kindle that aloofness, her indubitable independence and her 'get off' attitude. So many little characteristics which make them different to us! How else could I concoct a version of 'I don't love the vet' characteristics without being able to study my little feline role model?

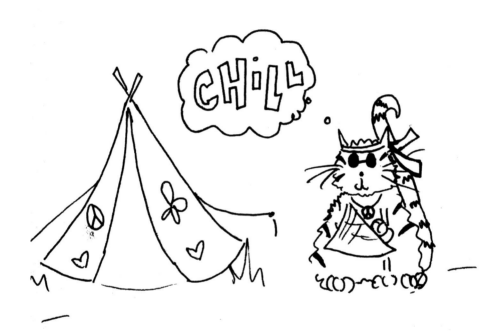

'All I want for Christmas,' said the puppy dog

So goes the song 'All I want for Christmas is me two front teeth!'

Try telling that to a very small yorkshire terrier called Babe, who, only weighing in at 1.5 kgs certainly deserves her title, even though she is all grown up (seven years old), she is so tiny that everybody thinks she is a puppy.

Continuing our Christmas theme, the tune referred to above keeps going through my head amongst others. So it was particularly apt that Babe should be brought in by a very nervous mum for an extensive dental procedure on Wednesday of this week.

I think because of her diminutive size, Babe receives a few more 'Ooos' and 'Ahs' than most, but it also means we have to go very carefully with the anaesthetic regime.

Babe's problem was that over several years her little 'teggies' had developed a copious collection of scale and associated gum damage, leaving her mouth in a rather anti-social state. A lick from Babe would spoil the beginning of a beautiful relationship, which sadly is an all too common fact about our companion pets.

Similarly the frequent concern of owners about their pets enduring a general anaesthetic for a teeth clean-up had stopped her owner broaching the subject with me for a couple of years, but now something had to be done because sadly, I was assuming that Babe was about to loose her front teeth, and a few more besides.

In fact, during her operation we removed twenty of her teeth, leaving only four in place (Please! Please! No letters from the experts out there asking why she didn't have the regulation 42 teeth in the first place).

Now you must not be worried by this revelation of huge dental extraction. It's sadly all too common because we dog (and cat) owners don't spend much time checking the dentition of our pets: all too frequently thinking nature will do the job - which it does not.

Anyway Babe will be fine. Her little gums will heal and she will be able to eat perfectly well, and will be much healthier, with a better life expectancy after removal of infected tooth roots – her Christmas turkey will taste sweet.

In the afternoon, Sally, our evening receptionist continued our Christmas theme. She regularly carries small animals around with her in the afternoon which have been hospitalised, and Babe, being so small, was a natural for the job.

Sally even proffered that she was teaching Babe to work the computers, but she had to be referred to as 'Santa's little helper' in my book.

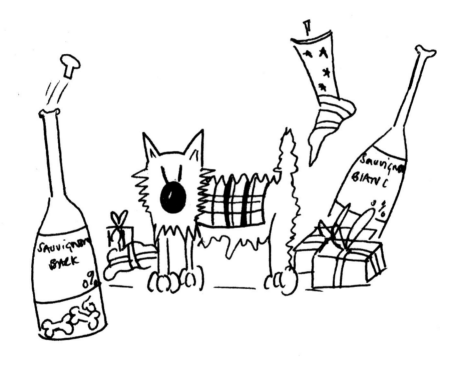

Cats with no fear of technology or toasters!

Picture this! I'd gone on a home visit to our local Woodland Cat Rescue. They were all down with some horrible virus (the humans, not the cats).

So they couldn't bring the ailing felines in to me.

I thought it would be funny to wear a protective face mask when I got there and, indeed, it produced the required laugh as I entered. But nowhere near the 'hoot' I produced as I stared into the conservatory to see a pair of wheels trundling around, attached to a very large cat!

I knew immediately that I was seeing one of these 'canny' orthopaedic support devices used to enable animals to exercise with paralysis of hindlimbs, and I have to say that it's something I don't particularly like. It's a personal thing. I can't get to grips with quality of life being assured in this way and, frequently, the incontinence that comes with such chronic injury makes for a difficult compromise.

But I have had to eat humble pie on more than one occasion, and a large slice was about to be shoe–horned in with voracity!

This cat, named Tyson, had suffered a fairly recent road traffic accident, rendering his hindlimbs useless, and a dysfunctional bladder, so a clever individual had produced a 'Tyson-mobile' from tubular steel and supportive straps, to which this duck had taken to the water with aplomb.

He careered around, turning on a sixpence, protecting his manor with ferocity, advancing toward other cats with crouched front legs, allowing the spectre of the trolley following behind to frighten the wits out of any brave enough to take him on – a veritable chariot of fire! Which Tyson uses to full advantage, and despite twice daily emptying of the bladder, he functions perfectly well and genuinely appears to enjoy life. Ok! He will not return to the life of his youth - a barn cat, controlling the local population of small furries, but my goodness! He really does appear to have plenty of fun.

That evening my wife related another adaptation of human technology by a cat. Cheeky, a cat belonging to my parents-in-law, has been doing his number ones all over their house for some time, and they have tried every trick in the book to break this bad habit, with little success. This has come about because he is disliked by all the other cats in the house, despite his gentle demeanour.

He had just decided that the kitchen toaster was an as yet untried haven to attempt some 'stress-busting'. Mum-in-law caught him at it, but was distracted by something happening in the garden before clearing up the mess, so she left to investigate.

She returned a couple of minutes later to find father-in-law, absent-mindedly munching on a round of 'well-flavoured' toast, piping hot from the abused machine. It was too late to prevent him eating the whole thing. Cheeky was nowhere to be found! My mind tinkered with the thought of what might have happened had the bread-burner been plugged in during his administrations!

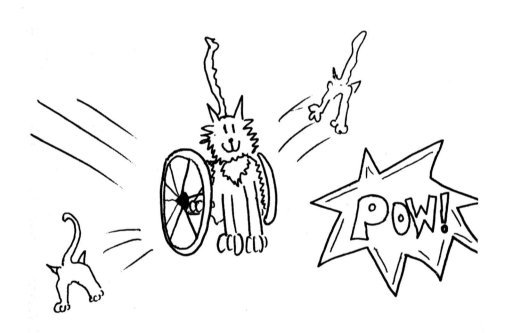

Pru's close shave with the surgeon's knife

Having three dogs and four cats should prepare me for regular visits to the vet: the laws of average would consider this likely.

Our youngest cat Jelly Bean received orthopaedic administrations earlier this summer when she fractured a hindlimb, so I thought it a bit unfair when I received a worried phonecall from my wife a few days ago, just as I walked into the practice, having left home five minutes before, reporting that Prudence, our oldest lhasa, was unable to walk on her hindlimbs!

When I examined her, her left hind was sticking out at an unusual angle, and she seemed to be in some pain.

These symptoms progressively worsened during the morning, even after anti-inflammatory drugs by injection, and by midday she was virtually paralysed.

X-rays showed some spinal disc degeneration, which was causing acute pressure on her spinal cord – something I had thought a likely problem considering the way she has always bombed around, and particularly highlighted as a concern when she regularly threw herself through the catflap at high speed.

Now my dilemma was what to do! Leave her to rest and hope for a slow return to normal? Operate on her myself? Or refer her to a specialist orthopaedic facility for surgery?

Only three choices. What luck! I mused.

A colleague suggested referral. My family wanted me to operate, and I, after a full appraisal of all the information, did nothing!

I plumped for cage rest. Not that the other options were wrong or unlikely to give her a good chance, but I was following my hopefully well-informed gut reaction, and yet again I personally witnessed how it must be for so many of my clients trying to make the correct decision about how best to deal with sickness and surgery on their own pets, when faced with a mass of medical jargon!

The more you learn, the luckier you get, and Pru slowly, but surely began to improve. At first very little of her back-end seemed to work, and then, quite suddenly she could do her ones and twos without help….the wiring appeared to be spluttering back into action!

The sticky–out left leg got stronger until she could stand on her own. Then of course she had to get clever and try to run, which was hilarious to watch but caused her pride a painful bump as both legs proved a little too rubbery.

Most recently she can walk and trot reasonably well, even though little wobbles appear from time to time, and straight lines consist of a series of veering curves.

She'll be home soon, bossing everyone as usual. My next dilemma? To plan how to stop her using the catflap. My wife suggests moving house to somewhere where we don't need a catflap – anything for Prudence, of course.

But as I always say 'If you fail to plan then plan to fail'….. I simply won't give her one of the special transistors to open and close the electromagnetic catflap that I will install shortly. Then of course I will have to deal with potential injury from a small dog hurling herself at an unforgiving catflap door……which page of my surgery book gives that information????

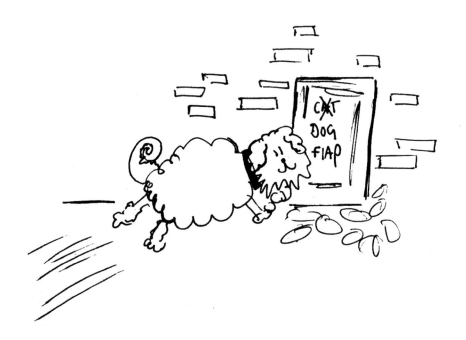

In praise of the three-legged cats

I would like to tell you about 'legs', but to be more precise, a lack of them! The pet which suffers from a deficiency of limbs perhaps fills an owner with trepidation, but I can tell you that of all the many animals who have been so badly damaged that amputation of a limb has become necessary, not one has failed to cope with its handicap so well that they became rather special.

I have had to amputate two badly damaged limbs this week, and I feel these little characters deserve a special mention, in the hope that our pet-owning public will perhaps look upon them as worthwhile to adopt or to persevere with, because despite being somewhat deficient in the leg department, they always seem to develop wonderful characters.

A couple of weeks ago, I mentioned one such cat named Breagha (gaelic for beautiful), a little tortoiseshell cat, unwanted by her owners when the extent of her severe back leg injuries came to light. In short, her amputation went well, and she began to convalesce so rapidly that she was rehomed within two weeks! I actually managed to con mother-in-law into having her, involving a small deception, of which she regularly reminds me!

At her new home, a couple of days of insecurity were followed by her completely taking over, deciding that she would sleep in her owner's bed, receive attention on demand, and eat whichever meal she desired, whenever she wanted. It's almost as if her invalid status had given her extra confidence in dealing with humans and other cats.

She can open doors by pushing both feet under the threshold and pulling hard; she specialises in tunnelling into anything and under all rugs, and can jump as normal, using her only hind limb as a form of spring, tripodding around at high speed and balancing on chair backs as if she is totally normal. Nothing escapes her curiosity. In fact, her new owner nearly jumped out of her skin when she went to the bag of cat food, only to find Breagha quietly sitting in the bag, attempting to nosh her way through fifteen kilograms of dry food.

As for the other cats! They have all been put in their place. She has taken over a radiator hammock owned by the tough guy of the household. It is as if they recognise an inner strength and power that this curious little cat retains like the writing through a stick of rock! Even the labrador dog has been utilised to full effect, as a comfortable, warm cushion, providing protection from the other cats when they cut up rough.

So don't fear! A three-legged cat will not let you down. I have seen so many who have lived a full life and provided their owners with endless pleasure, mainly because they become special. And don't just consider the regulation four legs – three can be just as much fun.

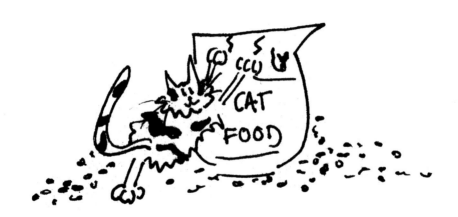

For my friend, 'Hercules'

A man stood on the roadside, just outside Carters builders yard at eight-o-clock on Christmas morning two years ago and, as I drove past, on my way up to the clinic, I slowed down, drawn by the desperate, searching look upon his face.

I stopped, and called out, 'Have you lost someone?'

'Well, I have. Our little Hercules went missing last night. Have you heard anything?' the man replied.

'I think I might have him up at the clinic. Follow me up there.'

The little bedraggled dog delivered to me by an anonymous Samaritan late on Christmas eve night, after he had nearly run him down, was in fact owned by the worried man, and when 'washed up' proved to be Hercules, renowned for his wondrous performances in the consulting room!

So began a lovely friendship with a super little dog and his lovely owners.

In all the years that I knew him, he was the finest patient, standing absolutely still for me to examine, never complaining or showing dissent towards my administrations. So he became one of my firm favourites, helped by a generous bottle of sherry, which he delivered personally each subsequent Christmas.

Sadly, he contracted a vicious form of viral hepatitis about a year ago. His blood biochemistry suggested that he would not survive. But without complaint, he stayed in the hospital for a week, then decided to get better and go home. Yet another dangerous, life-threatening experience overcome - he was a marvel!

Last Saturday night. Or should I say early Sunday morning, he became ill again. Yet again, it was very serious. A condition called pancreatitis, where the pancreas swells, sometimes so seriously that death is very sudden.

I had never seen Hercules so poorly, even with his hepatitis. He was groaning with the severe pain. There was no time for me to play with his name, as I always did, speaking to him in a French accent, calling him 'Eeercule'

He had every treatment possible. His worried mum and dad had to be sent home - there was nothing they could do!

Even with all his suffering, and heavy doses of drugs to control his pain, he lay still, uncomplaining, staring hopefully at me.

A few hours later, as I sat with him, he let out a gentle gasp and gently passed away. Nature had had its way.

Sadly I knew from the beginning that I could not save him. I was sad that my instincts proved right, because I had lost a good little friend. His family had lost a companion who had seen them steadfastly through some tough times. We will all miss you, 'little man'.

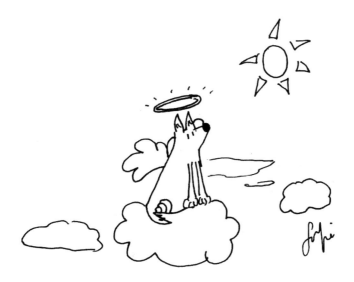

Guinness changes his mind about the carpets

It is not unusual to hear a client, who I know to be extremely house proud, talking with smiles and laughter about the damage caused to bespoke chattels by a new feline addition to the family, as it sharpens claws, and territory - marks the new environment.

We would keel-haul any human causing so much mayhem, but we all generally smile benevolently, and continue to discover hundreds of pounds worth of damage due to feline claws.

Our house is little different! Jelly Bean, our baby cat has a particular liking for the leg of the breakfast room table. It looks as if it's been gnawed by an alligator, rather than a few kilos of cat. But my wife, 'Protector of the cat universe', simply pulls the table cloth down a few inches rather too regularly, covering the damage and hoping that the leg gives way while I'm out.

Upstairs, things are much the same, where our 'heavy' (in physique and spirit) cat Guinness, has devastated the carpet edges of every bedroom threshold. You see, he has a complete hatred of closed doors, and shows his displeasure for such by plucking up the carpet edges and stripping them bare.

A few months ago, eldest daughter gratifyingly tripped with a tray of coffees and threw them headlong onto the upstairs landing. Oh dear!

No trip wire, honestly, which nice Mr. Insurance man believed, and kindly replaced new for old... I awaited Guinness's attack!

None came! I even watched him today staring intently at a closed bedroom door, willing it to open, but then turning on his heels and rushing headlong to beat ten bells out of the landing scratch pole – then returning to quietly stare at the door. I would never have believed it. At last a house-proud cat.

Scratch poles are placed strategically around our house to deliver some respite to the furniture. It's interesting to note that claw sharpening and territory marking by scratching at things are recognised as distinct behavioural entities. Our scratch poles have achieved this downstairs, but not until now, upstairs.

Back to Guinness. He eventually lost interest in his door and popped out for a quick 'barney' with the neighbour's tabby - saw him off with aplomb, and ten minutes later was found staring intently at the same door!

This time he didn't go back to his pole, but saw me sitting on our bedroom floor chatting. So he ran in and tested me out for scratchability, still looking with intense curiosity at his door.

I could hold on no longer. I took him and opened his door, whereupon he glanced into the room for the briefest moment and slowly wandered off downstairs. Why? I don't know. And why, a further ten minutes later he was performing another of his quirky games, which involves jumping into every conceivable small space in the house for about half an hour (even checking out the contents of the dirty wash basket), is beyond me - but why should I care? Our new 'deep pile' is as luxurious as the day it was laid. I love our new carpet almost as much as Guinness.

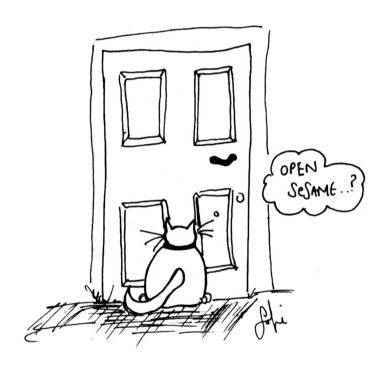

Have you ever been 'skunked'?

I suppose it's been said before, but I genuinely believe that God was not resting on day seven! He was busy creating the sublime vista that is Vermont, a small state squeezed into a small space below Canada and adjacent to the other New England states.

It's green, it's beautiful, and it's very, very quiet; filled with a convivial population of folk so unaware of crime and intolerance that you can leave your car unlocked anywhere, at anytime outside your house, which also requires no lock or bolt.

Indeed our friends Gerry and Ginny, with whom our family has just spent the past two weeks on our 'hols' do not know where their house keys reside, and they go on holiday leaving the house unlocked!

Where's the catch?… Well I don't think there is one unless, like me you spend a lot of time watching your pets. In Vermont, if you have four legs, things can happen to you which wouldn't in England.

Gerry's dog, Joey (a.k.a 'the wonder dog') had just been 'skunked' i.e spent a little too long fraternising with one of those well known black and white stinkers. I was called into the fray for advice but was totally unaware that a bath in vinegar is the best antidote to the pong.

Joe and his cat-partner, Renee, had also just been clipped. It helped remove some of Joe's smell, but I was amazed to see a little black and white cat scampering around with a rather aggressive 'number one' hairdo.

It transpired that during the summer, hair loss is so severe from domestic pets that clumps of it blow around on the wooden floors of all the houses in such volume that it gives the appearance of the tumbleweed, blowing around the proverbial deserted, one street, cowboy town.

Joe's fate paled as I met 'laid back' Clyde, an enormous St Bernard-cross, sprawled out in our friends air-conditioned offices, waiting for nothing in particular. Just managing to open an eye to acknowledge all the Ooo's and Ahh's of ourselves and visiting clients (had a bit of an ear infection that I couldn't help mentioning).

Then, while swimming in one of the huge, deserted lakes in the area we came across Lewis, a waggy, old retriever, who loved to swim out to anyone in a boat and accompany them back to shore. His owners felt that there was no need to pay them for his services! He even stood still in the shallows, allowing me to steady myself by holding onto his coat, as we disembarked from our rubber dingy – such manners!

Maybe Vermont isn't that bad after all if you're a pet! But then, at a barbecue one evening, Jenny (one of Gerry's daughters) was telling us about her spaniel and it's brush with the cold weather.

You see a lot of snow follows the gorgeous summers in this state. They had three metres of snow in March alone last year! And that little spaniel rushed headlong out into the fresh fall, chasing madly around until it came across some metal bars lying exposed to the intense cold and, you've guessed it, her first lick was her last. Her tongue froze immediately to the metal and stuck fast!

She survived the ordeal, but lost a layer of skin from her tongue, requiring soft foods for several weeks as it healed. I smiled and cringed at the same time, imagining the scene and the poor little dog's predicament.

Perhaps a few problems weren't ironed out on day seven after all?

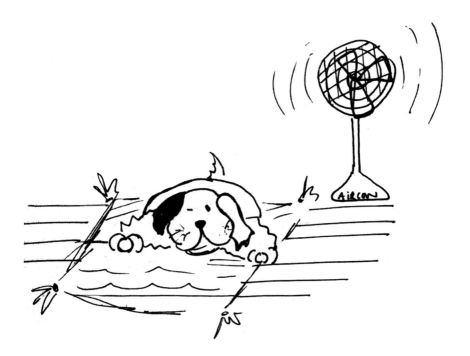

Zoo time at the clinic

I am often told by clients "You must enjoy your job"… I certainly do! I'm a lucky chap! I consider each day to be so different from the previous, that I could not begin to presume what will arrive in front of me on the consulting table each morning.

Today was remarkable in terms of the diversity of animals which we had hospitalised for treatment, and I would not expect to see another day like this for many a year to come. But I wouldn't be too sure!

As I walked along the cages, filling in the hospital sheets, it read more like Noah's ark than the vets.

A cockatoo with a fractured beak, sitting grumpily at the back of his cage, annoyed that the araldite fixing pins holding the beak parts together could not be pulled out because of a special head collar. An iguana beside it who had received a nasty 'chomp' from its long-suffering mate, requiring suturing.The owner made me laugh, because he felt she had deserved her 'chomp' because he had been to see me twice in the last fortnight with her male mate, injured by her during their little 'domestics'.

Next door sat a little lop-ear rabbit, very poorly, with a nasty bout of diarrhoea. I had to dose her with a special substance called a probiotic, which helps to settle the gut irritation in these little furries.

Sadly, the tiny hedgehog in kennel four was not responding well to treatment. He was admitted with severe unco-ordination, unable to stand or function properly, but this didn't stop him dragging himself twice-daily to a full plate of cat food, which he devoured without stopping. I have never seen one of these little animals eat so much. I feared for my cat food stocks when he became well! He had already gained 75 grams in four days, which was a 25% increase in his bodyweight.

A gerbil called Max was sitting mischievously in his little recovery cage, having had an infected cyst removed from the skin on his stomach. He appeared none the worse for his ordeal as he began to gnaw with real passion into the fresh toilet roll tube provided.

We often take in injured birds from the Broads in high numbers in the summer, and in the row of lower kennels sat the bedraggled set of those most recent arrivals. A pair of mallard ducks, weak and dehydrated from the effects of a severe bacterial disease called botulism, which affects many waterbirds when there is little rain and stagnant water areas proliferate.

Beside them sat a very poorly canada goose, recovering from the removal of fishing line from the lower part of one hind leg. And finally, a tiny little moorhen chick, separated from its mum, swam round in little circles, cheeping away, in its new, makeshift pond - a pale blue washing up bowl!

Where else could I have such fun in caring for animals?

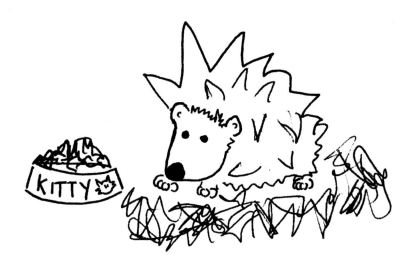

Getting Daisy's house in order

The two storey rabbit hutch seemed particularly difficult to move on Tuesday morning. It was stuck fast in the back of our four-wheel drive, and seemed destined to stay there.

It was the 'vital day' of the week i.e. **MY** day off. The weekend had been particularly busy and I was in need of a day to recharge the batteries, but here I was, yet again, doing something 'animal'.

'Pull it and lift a bit harder,' my wife advised.'It is for Daisy, come on!'

I acknowledged; pulled a bit harder and the hutch popped out.

Then my mother-in -law joined in, 'Could it just go over there, a bit closer to the pond?'

Of course it could. When all said and done. It was for Daisy!

Daisy stood by, quacking in her normal advisory manner. You see, she had every right. She is the matriarch of all the ducks on the pond. An Aylesbury 'waddler' of extreme proportion, saved from the duck farm with her devoted mate, Dandy; and saved yet again, because they were attacked by the residents ducks of another pond, then brought to me for nursing.

I became involved, treating their numerous head and eye injuries several months ago. They then became residents at 'the parents' pond, and bumbled around rather like Derek and Mavis from Coronation street, looking important, but having little overall 'duck power'.

Daisy laid eggs all over the place, regularly forgetting where they were, while Dandy proudly congratulated her efforts. Sadly, none ever hatched - a devoted, but unlucky set of parents.

Then, horror of horrors, a week ago, Dandy wandered onto the road, and was killed instantly by a speeding motorist.

We were all devastated, but in no way compared to Daisy. She mourned his loss for days, paddling about, quacking in what can only be described as a forlorn manner. It seemed vital to cheer her up, hence the rabbit hutch, which I was to convert into a 'duck hutch', for her and her friends, and then begin a search for a new mate.

We shouldn't have bothered! Within a week nature had cured her sorrow. A dapper little Mallard, called Humphrey had been installed as her new 'amour'.

Though only half her size, he struts manfully beside her as she goes about her business. Eggs are now being laid in haphazard fashion yet again and, life for now, has returned to normal on the pond... Just excuse me while I get on with the decoration of the hutch. Daisy seems to think that I'm slacking.

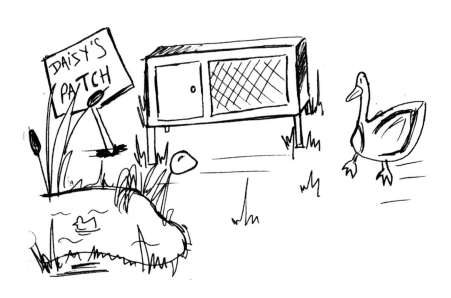

My welcome slice
of daily bread

Forget everything you've seen on television about how veterinary practice works! It's better than that!

Today, I had a wonderful morning surgery. A mix of lovely pets, interesting problems and, above all, fun as well. This mix of 'goodies' deserves some explanation so, while those more unfortunate in their work place signed papers, tapped into computer screens or sold things, let me explain what I was doing.

On the dot of nine, Ben came in for his annual booster. He's a bonny border terrier, who determines to lick you, whichever position you are in. Who do you know who would say 'thankyou' as you gave them an injection with an inch long hypodermic?

He was followed by dear old Stanley and Walter, two lovely black labradors, requiring Kennel cough vaccination: a vaccine which has to be squirted down the nose - what an unholy procedure! During which the owner and I frequently receive a good dose of protection as well!

Barney, a constipated cat, arrived shortly after. He had to be taken in for an x-ray to see what was causing such a severe gut upset.

Bobby Fisher was next. The gamest of yorkshire terriers, who suffered a 'Gazza' injury ie. A ruptured cruciate ligament in his knee. He has realised that three legs are as good as four, so the bags of rest required is being reasonably strictly adhered to. I accused his owner of playing football a little too aggressively with him. She, as a senior citizen, denies this vehemently.

Munchies, a small, eight week old kitten, bounced in for vaccination, but left dejected. A flea infestation, ear mites and mild flu symptoms meant a delay for treatment before inoculations.

Patient number seven was rushed in and out (owner late for a dentist appointment with her son). Sometimes you can't take time with a client, even if you wanted to!

A stabilized diabetic cat, suffering from hypothyroidism as well, came in at twenty past ten. Tom is a lovely old fellow. His owner has steadfastly learnt to cope with the daily injection of insulin. I'm convinced that Tom cringes each time she comes up to him with a gentle, slightly nervous hand, holding that syringe which saves his life every day!

A harsh cough heralded Sapphire's arrival – a dose of kennel cough we thought! She hadn't been in kennels which just goes to show the quirkiness of disease names.

Oscar and Benson calmly accepted their fate of vaccination. These two persian cats lay, like enormous furry carpet slippers, accepting with little more than curious scowls, the interruption of their rather lazy day.

Mr Bracher discussed his return to good health after a nasty hip fracture, while Jamie, his faithful westie, demanded his usual hug from me. I call him 'the mountaineer' because of his constant attempts to sit on my head! Jamie that is!

Eleven-o-clock, and gasping for a 'cuppa', but Dora, my final patient, was having none of it! As I searched through a mass of pearly-white, slightly kinked hair, I knew there was a rabbit in there somewhere. Her owner and I laughed about her rather rapid growth rate over a relatively few months. I consoled her by suggesting that regular combing of this slightly larger angora rabbit, might provide her, eventually, with enough fur for that elusive jumper.

Great animals - interesting owners, and such variety! That's what gets me up in the morning!

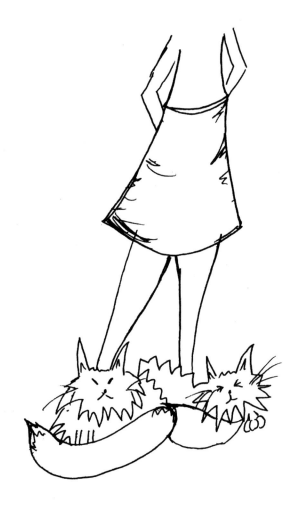

This was a sick parrot joke

It said on my computer that the next client was bringing in a 'Sick lor'. Which was a pity, because it should have said 'Sick Lory'. Sadly, my computer screen only has eight letter spaces in the box, which allows our receptionist to give the vet a short description of the illness for which the client's pet is appearing on waiting list.

This has led to several wonderfully descriptive terms appearing on the screen, but for now, 'Sick Lor' was the deal.

Having called in the owner, I realised that this was not, in fact a new Outer Mongolian illness, but a Lory, a small parrot-like species of bird, originating from Indonesia, and about a foot in body length.

It was a beautiful deep, velvety crimson in colour, with green wings, yellow bands on those wings, and purple-green on the tail. I was so transfixed by it's lovely colours that I failed to ask about it's exact name, rather discussing how beautiful these birds are, and trying to elicit some history about the ailment!

It transpired that the bird had belonged for many years to an old aunt, who had sadly died over the new year period: the new owner was a niece, who had promised to look after the little bird under all circumstances!

'So what's the problem ?' I asked, concentrating on the shining plumage, watching as well for any signs of ill-health.

'He's so sick, Mr Roe! He keeps shouting with pain, and when I go near him, he starts to roll over and over in agony.'

'But he looks so well. Is he eating ok?'

'No, he tries to eat, but can't swallow the food properly. It keeps falling out of his mouth. Poor love !'

I looked on. Not believing that such a healthy looking bird could possibly be so ill! Then the penny dropped, 'What sort of Lory did you say he was?'

'I don't know,' the client replied.

'Give me moment, please,' triumph sounding in my voice.

A quick flick through my exotic foreign birds book confirmed my suspicion. This was a Chattering Lory - no less: a species of small parrot well known for a harsh voice and persistent screaming when kept in an owner's living space, and not in a cage, particularly through the winter months. Caging seems to confine the rowdy behaviour. The rolling around and dropping food were simply bad behaviour, brought about by years of indiscipline, with, I presume, no obedience training (parrots can be very easily trained with word command and repetitive reinforcement). And now the little devil was playing the same games with it's new owner – poor little 'Sick Lor'!

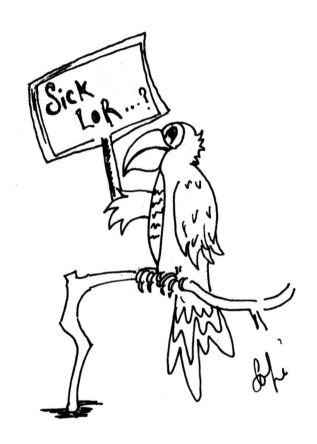

The luck of Mitzi Lawson

Mitzi is a little, female, tabby cat of indeterminate age, who you could only describe as retiring. She would normally shy away from visitors and look upon someone with a new car or delivery van as interesting, but to be watched from a distance.

So quite why she vanished so suddenly on that fateful Friday in early February is a complete mystery. A delivery van had brought new furniture to her home, and after that she was not seen again.

All the usual searches were made: at the local farm, along the roadside verges and dykes, and eventually the local vets – vain hope beginning to set in, rather than a practical answer.

The delivery man was called: attempts made to locate his drop-off points; notices were put up, giving information about a lost cat .

What was also so worrying was that she had no teeth and usually required careful feeding to survive. It all started to look so hopeless – no response from any of the charities, rescue homes, vets and numerous posters pinned up all over Norwich and central Norfolk.

Two weeks on, and she was given up as lost for good. Her owners vowed not to replace her. Her loss was so painful. I tried to give some support, but I could see in their eyes the strain of confronting the constant mental battle of what her fate may have been.

A month later (the grief settling a little), Mitzi began to be remembered for all her quirkish ways. The jokes about her ability to give you a 'nasty suck' with her vindictive gums became common place, and we all began to smile a bit more, vowing to prevent the same thing happening again!

Then, five week after her loss, a little cat was brought into the clinic from Woodland Cat Rescue, who live just round the corner from us. She had been with them since the 26th February. The vet who looks after the weekend calls commented on her lack of teeth, while the history of her being found near Fifers Lane, and being fed by a local Samaritan, seemed like a normal stray story.

Then the penny dropped! Mitzi's owners had rung Woodland to report her loss, clutching at any straws available: and now they had put events together, returning the complement – and yes, it was Mitzi!

The van driver was the unwitting culprit. He lived close to where Mitzi was found, and obviously she had (completely out of character) jumped onto his van and taken a fifteen mile journey into Norwich after the delivery, somehow escaping and living rough.

What is so remarkable is that all that time she was just a few minutes away from the clinic, and finally ended up living just round the corner at our local rescue society for a week. So eventually she was reunited, exactly thirty five days after going missing - what luck! Several lives lost over this one, I think; while my mother-in- law, who had lost her in the first place, will tell you that she had never given up hope!

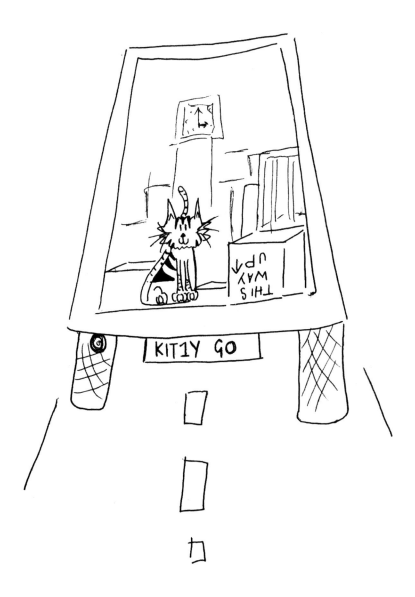

Midwinter madness in the snow

When it snows in Norfolk, we always complain about the traffic snarl-ups, and the poor state of the roads, as well as strange driving behaviour etc. But I think driving carefully and slowly has great benefit in such conditions; having had the pleasure of a four-wheel slide down Drayton hill, and coming down the steepest part of Ringland hills backwards a few years ago in snow conditions, while pursuing the course of my duties as a vet rather too rapidly.

Perhaps snow induces strange activity in many of us in our county, because when it snows there is always a flurry of strange behaviour from our beloved clients.

A client paged me at exactly 2.27 am this morning. It said so on my alarm clock!

In the usual fashion, I rang them back; asked relevant questions and advised an immediate visit to the clinic as it was a small pup that had had diarrhoea for about three days.

Sleepily, I de-frosted the car, and gingerly drove up to the clinic to await my visitor.

On the way, I asked myself what sort of fool was out in this weather. Sadly, it was only me.

I sat huddled up in the reception, waiting and waiting for all of forty minutes. No client arrived, so I rang the original number, hoping to find out where they were... No reply suggested they were on their way. So I waited for twenty minutes more, before ringing again - still no reply!

In the end, I went home - cold and somewhat annoyed, yet still somewhere inside me was a nagging concern that perhaps they had gone to the wrong place, broken down, or whatever.

The following morning, I rang the same clients to enquire about the preceeding evening, to be told that they had decided that venturing out in such icy conditions was not sensible, and they had disconnected the phone in case I tried to ring later on!

To say I was stunned understates the emotion that I felt, but it made me think about how people perceive normal behaviour. It is not unusual, when it snows for the odd client to ring to cancel their appointment, but then ask for us to visit because they dare not venture out onto the dangerous road!!!

My week went from bad to worse, when a dear old gentleman of about eighty five threatened to beat me up because a local charity had been unable to give him the voucher which he had gone to collect while it was snowing! Luckily, I was able to promise him that we would sort it out, and anyway, I could run faster.

I hope next week is a bit less fraught, but over the week-end, I'll think about whether I'm missing something. Perhaps I need to re-tune myself for that first winter flurry of snow?

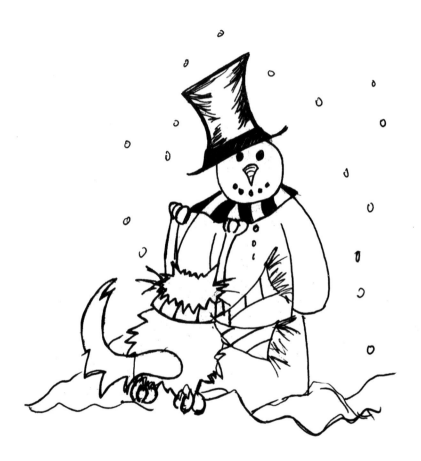

What is your cat up to at night?

It's that time of year again! The sun has been shining. Valentines has passed by, and our female cats begin to think of 'love'.

I tell all my clients that I would like a pound for every time I have been called at some unearthly hour by a distraught client, thinking that their little queen was dying painfully, from some form of poisoning, rolling round the floor in agony - screaming her last.

Thankfully, she is most often only suffering from the desire to mate.

Mrs Brown was one such client, who annoyingly thought it a huge joke to announce, 'Bet you can't guess who I am?' whenever she rang on the emergency service. It mattered not one jot if it was 3am or 3pm - always the same introduction.

After a few calls, I did indeed know who she was! But on this particular occasion she caught me out. The phone rang. I picked it up.

'Hello, Tim Roe, the vet speaking. How may I help you ?'

A growling noise, reaching to a primitive scream told me it was not one of my normal clients.

'Hello! who is this?'

'Listen! she's doin' it now.' replied a woman's voice.

More growls, more screams!

'Listen! I'm putting the phone near her now......Go on, my little darlin', do it for the vet,' she continued.

'Hello! who is this,' I asked, slightly more demanding in tone.

'It's me, and Tibby's in real pain...listen!'

The owner wouldn't tell me who she was; the screaming animal couldn't, and 'It's good to talk', wasn't a well-used slogan at that time .

'Well! she gone and stopped now,' the mystery woman continued, 'She's lickin' herself. I'll ring ya back if it happens again.' The phone went dead!

'Bet you can't guess who I am?' began to materialise in my mind.

So, dear reader, or client. First and foremost, please tell your vet who you are, and secondly, fear not the little female cat screaming, apparently in agony, at some strange hour of the night, bobbing her tail up and down, and rolling around. She may just be coming into season, particularly at this time of the year, when females reaching puberty at 7-12 months of age start to cycle, preparing to mate.

The reproductive behaviour can be particularly intense around February to April,and again June through to July; sometimes a third phase occurs in September and October. Watch out for the explosion of the strange signs described when the queen comes on 'heat'. It can last 3-6 days, and end as abruptly as it started.

So there we have it!- but a word of caution! Please remember that your female cat can have 2-3 heats during each of these three periods of activity. That means that most of them, if left to mate freely, could deliver two litters to you each year, averaging four kittens a time.

We certainly have enough unwanted little kittens at our surgery each year, as do the local cat rescue societies; so, please, do consider having your young cats neutered (male and female) to prevent the soaring problem of unwanted litters. Please do not hesitate to contact your local vet for advice regarding female cats behaving unusually at this time of the year. They would prefer to reassure a worried owner on all occasions, and if anyone requires further information on any of the above they can contact myself, or any member of staff at Willow veterinary clinic in Hellesdon.

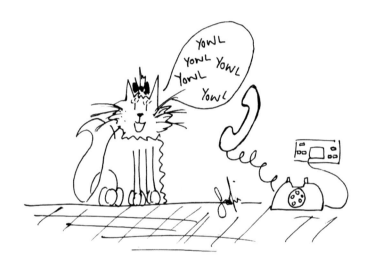

Are the fat cats happy?

There was an air of relief in the practice this week: the last box of chocolates, generously given to us by our clients at Christmas, was finally eaten and laid to rest, so all the female members of the clinic began to re-affirm their promises of careful dieting, laxed as they had become after New Year resolve.

I have to admit that I achieve a generous level of contempt from all of them, as I ignore my stomach line and indulge in copious calories, teasing the looks of desire that such a carefree, reckless attitude achieves.

But one person seeking advice about an obesity problem stumped me this week, when she brought in her 17 year old cat who I have treated for the past eleven years, and who is as fit as a fiddle, climbing a six foot fence with ease, and 'seeing off' every neighbouring cat and stranger with the same enthusiasm as seen when a youngster.

"Oh, I don't think she's very happy," said the owner, with concern.

"Why not?"

"Well, I think her weight is a bit of a problem."

"But, she weighs eleven kilos! And has done for all of the time that I've known you both. So why has it become a concern now?"

She began to whisper, and it transpired that she suspected that the cat could no longer get round to lick it's bottom because it was so fat, preferring to drag it along the carpet!

I lifted the tail to check on two little glands that reside in that region, called surprisingly, 'The anal glands' and, as suspected, I found them impacted - the cause of the whole problem! But as I turned, triumphantly, to report my findings, still holding the tail up in the air, the cat forcefully emptied those glands expertly in my direction, a foul splodge ending up in my hair and an even bigger one went straight into my mouth, as I began to speak.

This is the second time in my career that such an auspicious event has taken place! The cat owner was crying with laughter! I held my face under the cold tap, trying to wash the horrible taste and aroma from target areas. My professional advantage in tatters. The cat stared, self-satisfied, out of the window - mission accomplished!

Would you continue with further advice on obesity in the domestic cat after such an episode?... I think not. And since I had been thwarted yet again in getting over any useful point about the cat's weight, I gracefully withdrew from the battle.

I continued to swallow down the fading flavour of rotten, dead fish, mixed with putrid meat (which describes cat anal gland contents in a nice way), regained some composure and feigned a slight smile for the client, who was still enjoying the joke immensely, bless her!

It is obvious that this story will pass into folklore, as many have done before, but I will stand by my attempts to offer dietary advice to all cat owners! Except to the restaurant owner in Thailand, who (this week) forgot to feed the tigers that he kept in a cage on his premises to entertain his customers. When he noticed his error, he entered their enclosure burdened with supper. The big cats were so pleased! They ate him first, and then their cat-meat for afters.

101

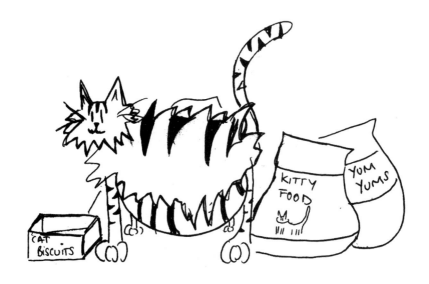

Deceived by a flying tortoise with attitude

The spring brings a regular influx of tortoises with a multitude of problems: most related to their explicable desire to live life in a Mediterranean climate rather than the changeable British one. Tortoises are not supposed to hibernate for huge periods: their bodies are much better suited to short ones – chronic frost, ice and chill are not in their database.

Add to this our evermore temperate climate over the last few years, and you can see why your average Fred or George is one confused reptile.

Tony, a forty-something beefcake has visited the clinic too regularly for his liking in the last few months: a victim of post-hibernation anorexia, demanding twice-weekly tube-feeding with Mr Roe's magic tortoise nectar: a concoction of baby food, a specialist multi-mineral and vitamin powder, a thing called a probiotic, to get his guts working; and a liquidised convalescent dog food.

Now 'big Tony' looks as fit as any well built chelonian could, but he refused to eat – point blank! I hospitalised him for a week. I gave him baths and trundled him round the garden in the sun. I even picked succulent dandelions to tempt him! Still no luck

He was fed as described, and took every stomach-tubing with mild manners. I even introduced him to playing pretend aircraft as I scooped him up from his owners and took him through for his meal. He became known as 'the flying tortoise'. It seemed as if he was enjoying it all a bit too much. I even suggested that his flying lessons and a power-packed meal twice weekly was making him rather blasé about eating for himself.

Eventually, I asked for a week off from his visits, attempting to hit home with his need to eat for himself. He hasn't returned! Duped by a tortoise?

Little George arrived hot on Tony's heels. A tiny five centimetre youngster, with little gangly legs and infected eyes. This looked like a lack of vitamin A, more commonly seen in fish-eating terrapins. He was essentially blind but still whizzed round our vivarium looking for the warm spots.

Again, I began a regime of tube-feeding while he was hospitalised, and regular vitamin injections, all somewhat harder to administer considering his minute size. One millilitre of liquid food filled every corner of his tiny stomach and, as I carefully computed a dose of vitamin A for a tortoise, the useful advice came to light that it should be between 10 and 15000 units, depending on size of the tortoise... pick a figure!

Thankfully, George suffered no ill-effects from the frequent injections and went home after a week, with the advice that his return to normal service would be slow. But what joy! I saw him last week and those little eyes are wide open, the legs are somewhat more solid and he will do well.

I'm just hoping that tortoise alert is over for another year.

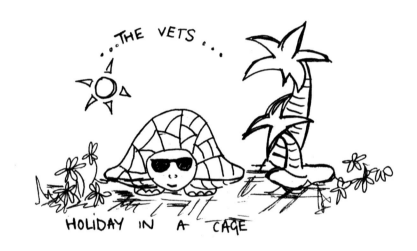

Please can I look inside your head?

Sometimes incredible things happen between two people. You must have had an experience which makes you feel as if someone has just looked inside your mind and seen your inner self? Or perhaps you have had your pet look at you in a way which made you feel as if your mind has been read? No!... well I have tonight: it happened with a dog called Bessie, who is the most delightful black and tan crossbred, and who has had x-rays recently to diagnose the severity of the arthritis affecting her elbows.

To cut a long story short, she has embarked upon a course of injections to help stem the deterioration of her poor old joints, regular painkillers and a crash diet!

What a blow! Nearly every pleasure in life reduced to a fraction of its former self. Tonight, her owner brought her in towards the end of evening surgery. I called them both in: Bessie stayed put, lying on the waiting room floor, staring straight ahead, concentrating on what she wasn't going to do.

I went out to get the special injection, leaving them time to sort themselves out, returning to find Bessie sitting on the consulting room table, waiting for me. As I walked into the room, she looked straight into my eyes. I felt as she was reading my mind; that she knew everything that I was thinking – and she kept doing it, until I mentioned it to the owner.

'She does it all the time!' he explained. 'She seems to know everything we are talking about at home and understands it all.'

It was remarkable – to feel as if an animal could pick up my intentions at will! It got me thinking about the frequent episodes in my working life when I have been 'second-guessed'. And I realised that it's more frequent than perhaps I perceive. Why?

I don't want to get into the semantics of E.S.P. and all that, but I truly believe that our pets have powers of understanding and premonition that we cannot begin to imagine. Why, for example, do so many cats go missing in the hour or so before being squashed into a cage and driven to the surgery?... because we either have a larger proportion than normal of clients who use it as an excuse for being late or, more likely, Kitty picks up our intentions, somehow.

Similarly, dogs are frequently reported as becoming anxious in the period prior to coming to the vets. So what is the answer? Well, it is well known that our pets spend much more of their waking hours watching us, than the other way around. It comes from the primeval need to survive by being aware of what the rest of the pride or pack is doing.

But, let's not get too scientific! Do you know what I really think? I truly believe that your pet can read your mind, not necessarily in the rational way that we might presume, but enough to sense a change in mood or intention.

Next time you bring your pet to the vet, think about it. Next time you feel a bit down, see if your pet changes his or her demeanour. Try to tune into your pet, because they are far better tuned into us than you can imagine. But don't be too clever in understanding. As another client warned me. 'If we did know how animals do it, someone would probably pinch it!'

But finally, don't believe me verbatim. Test this theory in this festive season. Look into your pet's eyes and ask them if they truly knew what you had wrapped them up for Christmas – or did they simply take a peek when you weren't looking????????

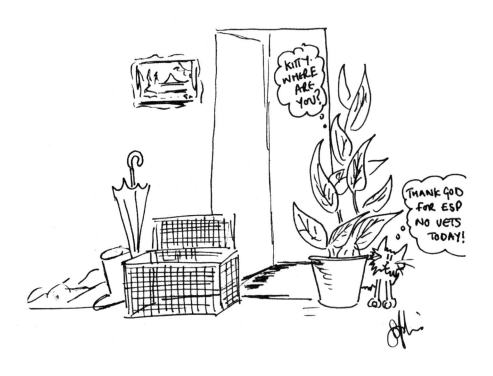

Treating the whole pet and nothing but the pet

It is becoming more apparent, day by day, that life is more complicated. Perhaps that's why we humans look for varied and sometimes unusual methods of coping with the stress and subsequent illness that our busy lives produce.

As this thought entered my mind, I was advising the owner of a lovely old retriever about the potential value of acupuncture to treat his pet's aggressive arthritis; even going on to mention the possibility of magnotherapy and homoeopathy as adjuncts to a holistic approach, then touching on diet and the use of probiotic-containing foods which might help the immune system.

You may be surprised, but 'holism' is everywhere. Treating of the whole being, including mental and social factors rather than just the symptoms of a disease, is fast becoming the most popular way forward for many sick humans and their pets. It is not the domain of the 'airy' individual who denounces convention: and this is proven by the fact that we all look to a much broader conception of health and well-being than we have ever done in the past one hundred years, using diet, relaxation technique, herbal treatments and a plethora of gizmos to help us, without resorting to a bottle of prescribed tablets or medicine.

It is particularly interesting to look at the use of veterinary diet to improve health and behaviour, ever since Roger Mugford, Britain's leading veterinary authority on behaviour, suggested that, in his research, the golden retriever and german shepherd were two breeds particularly sensitive to minor changes in food nutrition, hypothesising that years of in-breeding had in some way led to immunosuppression, which could directly affect behaviour!

Similarly, because the first duty to our patient is to attempt to control pain and/or any suffering, it is vital to realise that many dogs with behavioural problems can simply be suffering clinical pain.

Perhaps we should consider wider fields of treatment and diagnostics than ever before. I applaud the idea of animals with chronic pain being referred to a 'pain clinic', where osteopathy and chiropractice might be available alongside conventional drugs. Not only would it improve diagnosis but it would also show that veterinary medicine has a desire to broaden its horizons.

Inevitably, all my 'wofflings' meet with an exception to the rule. Badger, a four year old 'staffie' followed the old retriever into my clinic.

'What's the problem?' I asked.

Two little girls, accompanying a rather nervous looking father started to giggle.

'Well he's took to winding quite a lot,' said a nervous northern accent

'What!' I asked.

One little girl, about eight years old, could control herself no longer. She looked to her sister (I presume) whose giggles confirmed her waivering confidence. 'Mum says he won't stop popping from his bottom!' she announced.

I got the gist of it. Now exactly where do I begin the holistic approach to chronic wind?

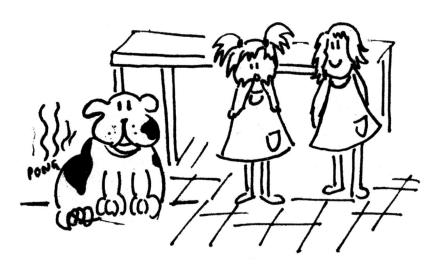

PONG

Everyone said 'Who loves ya?' – but it wasn't enough!

Spare a thought for stray cats as you read this article! It can't be much fun scavenging for a living – constantly being driven from one place to another, like some hobo, possibly confused by the mixed instincts of survival, frequently demanding a fearful response, and a waning memory of domestication

So it seemed to be another one of those cases of a cat's bad fortune when a little, half–starved tomcat was noticed by two of my clients while driving through Sprowston. They had to chase him pretty hard to catch him, but what they presented to me was a very sorry sight: a little fellow so emaciated that I could count every rib clearly and, worse still, he had virtually no hair due to a severe allergic reaction to fleas, which were eating him alive from head to toe!

He cowered on the exam table, moving in that slow-motion manner, so characteristic of cats, particularly when frightened or challenged by another feline.

Yet typically, this was not a preparation to attack me: he was just mighty scared! We all talked of what he must have suffered during his enforced wanderings. Appearing to be so shy and retiring, he must have had a tough time of it. So often strays are attacked in 'gang-like' fashion by the local feline mafia, sending them onto their next port of call.

But I wasn't down–hearted! As he tucked into a plate of cat food with gusto, I warmed even more to his insecurity. He kept looking round behind him, as if expecting to be chased off at any moment. The comfortable confines of his B & B kennel hadn't settled his anxiety yet.

The hearty meal was followed up by a less pleasant squirt of flea spray. I'd have him looking a million dollars in a few weeks. New hair growth; a little operation to curb his body odour problem, and we'd have him up in shining lights in the RSPCA rehoming parade.

We had even given him a new name! Kojak! Thoroughly apt considering his state of deficiency in the wig department. Yet I was sure that this little chap would sell himself with the 'hail-fellow-well-met' informality so commonly seen to develop in strays after a few weeks TLC! The baldness might even enhance the attraction to a willing prospective owner, and me bouncing around saying 'Who loves ya baby?' was just to get him used to his new title.

I had it all planned for the next day: speak to the RSPCA about his medical needs; blood test him for leukaemia and cat-aids; then send him on his way!

Everything went well. The RSPCA even had a place for him right away. Kojak filled his boots at breakfast yet again! Then I noticed the spot of blood on his nose. He began to sneeze more often during the morning, spraying droplets of blood all over his kennel.

I knew something was up! It was confirmed by the blood test. He was positive for feline leukaemia, a vicious viral disease so often carried and spread by activity of stray and feral cats which would, no doubt, cause his demise fairly soon.

I'd promised him so much. As I put him to sleep, I felt that humanity had let him down in some peculiar way. Nature couldn't help him either – he hadn't had a very nice life!

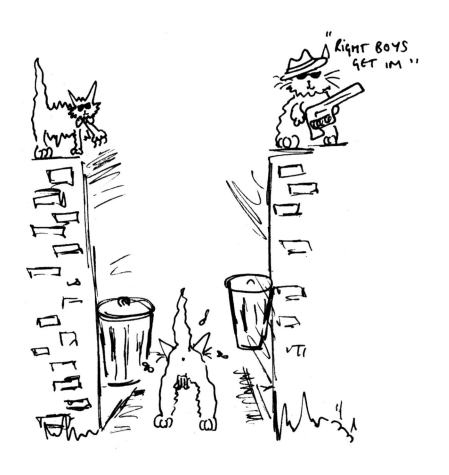

Hot chickens on the run

Plenty of people keep exotic pets these days, and I'm often asked to examine and treat those which, in times gone by, would only be considered as food providers. For example, the humble chicken is nowadays a frequent visitor to the surgery, exalted to the position of pet rather than livestock.

One of our good friends loved her hens. They were always known as 'the chickies'; tended with much love and care, and talked about as members of the family. We were constantly in their debt for a regular supply of the tastiest fresh eggs you could imagine, and frequently informed of their antics.

Then disaster struck. A fox was presumed the culprit of a vicious night-time attack upon the six layers, leaving four dead and two badly wounded!

I treated both those badly injured birds for several weeks: between us we tube-fed them regularly and one regained good health fairly quickly but the second survivor, a large rhode island red suffered a constant problem with a recurrent abscess due to bite wounds, which eventually led to the sad decision to put her to sleep.

Sadness purveyed the weeks following, but the remaining chicken endeared herself with a display of fine gardening skills, as she socialised with her human companion.

Several months passed - until this week the big moment came when the time was right to restock. We travelled in the sweltering heat to Weeting, a few miles from Thetford, to visit a wonderful chicken purebreed centre, where you are immediately surrounded by fluffball-chicks of all types, whizzing to and fro. Massive exotic Asian species like the brahma, the cocks strutting around doing a gangly frog march; and the poland, a small variety with distinctive foppish crests, which give them a look akin to animal versions of the Beatles.

I could have stayed all afternoon, looking at and learning about all these beautifully coloured and carefully bred birds, but 'the new chickies' had to be delivered to their new home.

I'd brought three wire cages for transport, to allow plenty of air flow and we set off with the car air-conditioning at full blast, while the four rhode island reds and two black astralorpe-hens burbled away in the back. As long as they kept up the noise I knew they were in no distress!

An hour later they were released into their new coup with an attached, small exercise area to allow acclimatisation, before being allowed full use of a large wilderness-run full of wild plants, and ripe for days of exploration.

We scattered a small trail of corn outside to entice them into the cool, grassy shade under the spread of hoary old apple tree, and within a minute or two an inquisitive wattle popped out of the side door, followed by a gentle 'peeping' noise - and then a chicken, recognising a meal when it sees it.

They all looked happy! Can chickens look happy? I'm not sure, but they'll be cherished and cared for like no others and I will be kept regularly informed of progress which considering my involvement with the grief of a few months ago will make me feel good!

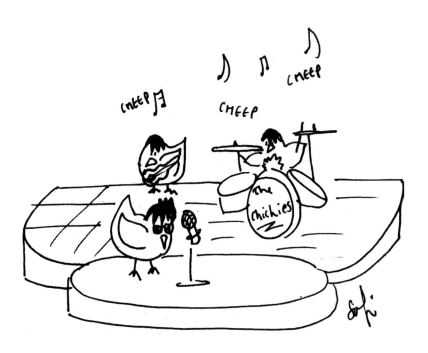

Providing the entertainment at the East of England show

I was just thinking how cavernous the boot of the beautiful Jaguar 'S' class appeared: you could probably get the contents of the millennium dome in there, I was musing, when a finger prodded me in the ribs.

I turned to confront a little boy who had spoken to me earlier, who said......! Well, I'll tell what he said a little later.

You see, I was at the East of England show, doing a little spot where the general public could come up to me and ask any vet question they wished. 'Sniper fire' rained upon me all day, as the gathered owners quizzed me.

I should have realised that someone (or more) would try to catch me out!

One gentleman came up, asking pertinent and well-informed questions about his dog which suffered from separation anxiety, where a dog left on its own becomes tense, stressed and frequently destructive.

It was not until I was halfway through my 'public flogging', that he owned up to the fact that he had already sought his own vet's opinion and that of an expert in canine behaviour. And then, in a loud voice reported to the assembled crowd that what I had just advised him was the opposite to the behaviouralist's.

Seeing my opportunity, I countered with, 'But you've just said that none of the advice has worked, so why don't you try my ideas and perhaps also try the anti-anxiety drug for dogs, called clomicalm?'

'Huh, I thought you'd say that,' he countered. 'That's what my vet tried to sell me, and I reckon that's far too expensive!'

'Has anyone else got any questions?' I said, moving quickly along.

That's when small, finger-prodding boy arrived. 'Oi, mister!' he bawled. 'My cat keeps going all wobbly! Why's that then?'

I benevolently turned him to face the audience, explaining likely reasons for his cat to be wobbly; quickly finding out that the cat was eighteen years old, so I made a small comment, 'If your granny was that old, she might be a little weak and wobbly. How old is your Granny?'

'I dunno!' he replied. But he left, looking happy with my advice and witty little comments.

So back to the Jaguar 'S' type and the rib-prodding episode.

The same little boy as above had obviously been deeply affected by my comment about his granny and had traced me to the Jaguar stand. I jumped up out of the car boot. He eye-balled me and announced, 'Oi mister, my granny is fifty eight, and she sez she's not wobbly at all!' With that he marched off.

That was just before I decided to go home!

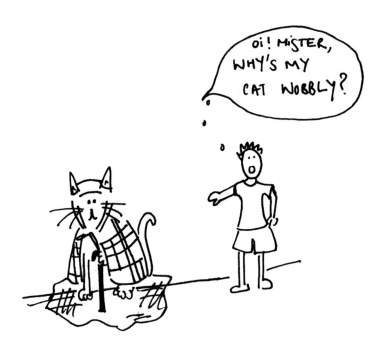

Snoops and Bess enjoying their twilight years

Should I say it? It is now thought that dogs have the ability to learn dominant behaviour much earlier in life than they would in the wild pack environment because of... us!

We are the weakest pack members that a dog could wish for and constantly give off messages to our beloved pets which suggest that we are the subservients and they are the bosses.

Believe me, it's true. You've only to hear an owner calling their dog a good boy when it's trying to bite me in the surgery to see how wrong we can get it: not deliberately I hasten to add, but because human language does not translate easily into 'doggy'

Thankfully our chosen companions for domestication do not take as much advantage of us as they might and, more often than not, will fit perfectly into our 'human pack', so will frequently behave in a way which befits comparison to us.

I did see two corresponding examples of dog behaviour at one clinic this week which left me wondering whether old-age quirkiness in our pets is closely comparable with that of humans.

I speak of Snoopy and Bess, two old seniors: both of whom dropped in for health checks, one after the other, this week.

Snoopy has severe heart problems, wobbly old legs and failing sight but the constitution of an Ox and a tail that wags for England.

During our conversation his owner related that they <u>have</u> to get up to him regularly during the night, as he wakes up and needs attention. We joked about old age and his uncanny ability to require this attention every couple of hours and, with a consistency that meant they all took turns to be on 'Snoop patrol', rather as young parents swapped nights in looking after babies that wake up during those first few months of life.

Snoops sounded to me as if he'd got exactly what he wanted, and more, because one member of the family regularly gets in from work at 2 am and has a play period with him as well.

Accusations of attention-seeking, and philandering during the day, in preparation for a busy night of waking up his owners were preferred, and denied.

But Bess, in for a re-check on tumour re-growth problems, supported my claim, for she was reported as <u>demanding</u> that her owner went to bed at 9pm every night. She sleeps on the bed, of course, and I could find no reasonable suggestion as to why a dog who has worked out that such a demand is accepted regularly by her owner should not continue to 'try it on'

The hypothesis that dogs behave in a manner related to a stimulus and response blows itself out of the doggy bowl with these two. They know exactly what makes them happy and exactly how to get it from we humans, pathetic pack members that we are!

Excuse me by the way for any spelling mistakes in this article. Hattie my little cavalier king charles has been sitting on my lap while I've been typing. It's been the only comfortable place in the house for the last half hour she tells me – how could I refuse?

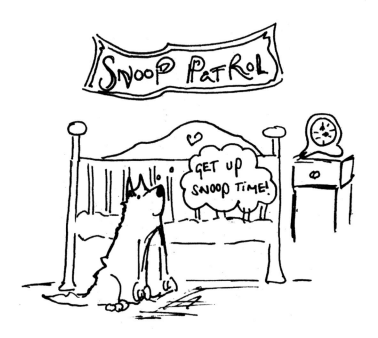

Super Sandy saves himself from serious surgery

You wouldn't think it possible that I would applaud 'small furries' such as rabbits or guinea pigs for courageous or sensible behaviour! They just are not those sorts of animal: cuddly, companionable and great fun, but not given to the sort of stoicism of other pets like dogs, who can tangibly display what appears to be great determination and bravery, and a smidgeon of common sense.

Well I am wrong! In the first instance, Sandy, a ten year old dwarf lop rabbit has conclusively proven me incorrect.

He began a long illness well over a month ago, when we noticed a rapidly growing abscess on the side of his face. These things are particularly unpleasant for them because they develop very aggressively, usually from a tooth root infection, producing persistent, encapsulated tissue damage, which normally requires extensive surgery for removal, and which frequently returns to cause more problems.

Enough of the mechanics of it all. Suffice to say that I never met a better, more compliant bunny in all my administrations! Initially I presumed things would go the way of most such infections; draining the abscess frequently, but ending up with such a poor response that we might have to give up hope – but no such thing! Sandy has been treated twice weekly for over a month, flushing the abscess, and packing the wound with antibiotics. And he has never complained. He sits still while I pull him around, squeeze the area, open up the wound to continue drainage, and then clean it up – what a guy! Descriptions of bravery abound from all involved. Most of his peers would have climbed the walls, but not him. And all this at an age when you might expect him to give up with all the stress. He is genuinely a courageous little fellow and, most important, the abscess is virtually gone!

Next in line for a gong from the 'pet palace' are Looby-loo and Floe: two exceptional guinea-pigs (belonging to Harriet, the best friend of my daughter Emma) who knocked me out with their display of behaviour at the week-end. As I said, it's unusual to think of these little beings being capable of displays of wisdom and common sense, let alone an understanding of human communication - but this pair defied all this.

I watched as they were removed from their run on the lawn. Their owner shouted to them to go to their cage. One behind the other, they trundled off across the grass, climbing jauntily up a set of stairs, then moved rapidly to sit beside a couple of flower pots, one guinea pig to a pot, where they waited to be picked up and lifted into their cage, whistling all the way.

I accused both of them of being clockwork versions of these little pigs, but No! they really are flesh and blood, and remarkably talented!

What can I say! Human attributes of bravery and common sense with wisdom uncommonly shown by small animals... what next? My wife says that this shows conclusively that it might be possible for me to be trained to remember exactly what it was that she sent me down to the local shops to buy.

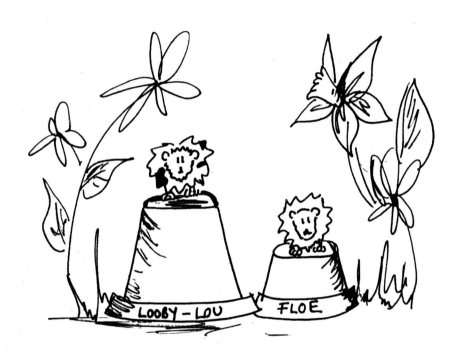

The official line on avoiding examination!

I am an expert! You pet dogs out there can use various techniques to avoid or disrupt a visit to the vet, and I know most of them. Therefore I am producing my official list of procedures used to foil him or her. I would appreciate full compliance in taking note of the following specific methods – and no passing this on to owners. What do they know!

Look surprised, on arrival in the carpark. Jump out in a relaxed fashion, but then pull very suddenly in the direction of the road. It might just fool your owner into taking you for a walk instead!

As you are enticed into the clinic, cock your leg up the wall. The vet might just sniff it and run away!

Pull immediately towards the chairs. A quick retreat under one of these might conceivably make him think you're not there... nice one !

As the vet calls your name, look shocked, 'What me?' you must appear to say. Then gently go with the owner's pull on the lead. Pretend that you are going in the right direction, then choose either a swift lunge for the door, which might just open at that moment to allow escape or, two feet from his consulting room, apply air brakes. Your owner will feel totally embarrassed, because everyone in the waiting room will laugh, and the vet may say something to make your owner wince like, 'Ho, Ho! I didn't know you two were the floor show, this evening.' Owner may then run away as well.

If there is no escape, and the consulting room door shuts behind you, then really go for it. Cock that leg, and simply open the flood gates; cover his floor until he looks really annoyed, and goes to fetch the mop. He's not much good at that, because he has people called nurses who usually do that. They don't get annoyed, so don't try this one with them. As he leaves, push through the gap and run for it!

If all of the above fails, then simply sit down recalcitrantly, making it as difficult as possible for him to examine you. If at all possible, do this in a corner of the room from which it is impossible to extract you without (at least) causing a mild back strain.

At all costs, appear at all times to be totally indifferent to any of his concerns. If you show willing, he'll probably stick another needle in you, and ask you to come back next week, with some lame reference to 'We must check his or her progress.' Don't trust this. They like prodding you! That's why they're vets.

When he's finished with you, he usually sits back, trying to be all light-hearted, making little jokes. Well don't be fooled! Stick your nose right at the door, making sure that he's aware you need to leave. That door will eventually open.

Hope that the bill is very high. That seems to prevent owners wanting to take you back very often!

Take this advice and all trips to the vet can be made a short as possible. Next week – cats get ready! Advice from a friend, to help you empty that surgery.

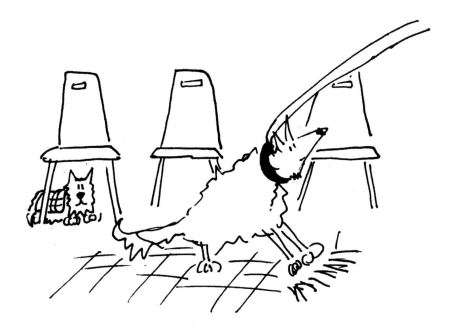

The stuff that kittens are made of

I'm not sure that it's quite fair that I am perceived as having almost magical ability in word and deed to diagnose and treat all manner of conditions in pets, who can neither describe their symptoms nor necessarily tell me how they feel. It's good then, that I am a persistent optimist!

I was reminded of this today when an owner described how he would suffer from illness himself for much longer without complaint (and without visiting his doctor) than he would allow his pet to be ill; and that he expected his pet to improve with treatment much more quickly than he would himself, with medicines provided.

It was unusual then, on the same day, to come across a little kitten, called Buzz, who seemed to give all of us at the clinic no feeling of optimism whatsoever! Even the owner had no expectation that he would survive.

This tiny little chap was so lifeless, dehydrated, anaemic and seemingly unable to eat. He had a harsh, rasping respiration and running nose. We all felt that it was hopeless! He was even too ill for us to get a small drop of blood needed to run some basic tests. He weighed just under half a kilo, and we felt we were likely to sit and watch him fade away.

But could we let our optimism be denied? We began to work out a regime of supportive measures to keep this plucky chap going. I think it was when he sat looking straight at me from his kennel, that I decided to get cracking, because when he looked me straight in the eye, mewed forcefully, without any sound, it felt as if he was telling me to get on with it!

During his hospitalisation, he was given special fluid support, force-fed liquid feed and then, when we managed to get that tiniest sample of blood, we found it full of fats which shouldn't have been there. Perhaps, sadly, the kitten had a developmental disorder which, being based in the liver, would prevent it from ever functioning properly.

But Buzz was having none of this! Within two days of beginning our therapy, he started to groom himself - a fantastic sign. Then he began to eat and produce perfectly formed little presents in his litter tray for us.

Each day he became stronger; and five days after being hospitalised, with no hope, he was sent home - still a skinny little thing, weighing only 550 grammes, but alive and determined to live.

At re-examination, a few days later, his weight was being maintained, with good feeding, but I still couldn't tell his owner what had gone wrong: none of our tests had thrown up a positive result for any specific condition, but in front of me was a kitten, getting better each day.

So I could not tell what was wrong. I couldn't treat a specific condition, and I still cannot tell the owner exactly what the future will hold. But somewhere, I picked up that kitten's determination to survive. Perhaps that's the 'magical' ability vets sometimes have! To mix optimism, clinical skills and the odd message from our patients, and hope that they give us the result.

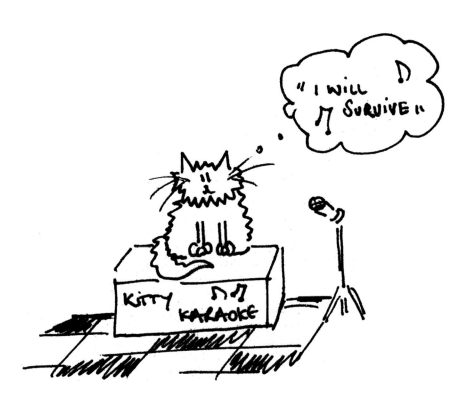

Convincing myself that I'm funny

We can, I am sure, all remember with fond affection the comments and one-liners that the much-loved Eric Morecambe delivered regularly to his sidekick, Ernie, whose mixture of surprise, lack of understanding and confusion, were as important in gaining the laugh

These little moments required no words of explanation. They were guaranteed winners; and we generally expected them while watching the show.

I have several very common 'guaranteed winner' comments which I use regularly to raise a smile (and sometimes to be a tiny bit mischievous), such as my very own favourite, when palpating the abdomen of a pregnant bitch, proceeding to announce to the client the presence of a successful pregnancy, followed by something like, "And it's two boys and three girls!"

The client looks amazed, and yet again I have succeeded in amusing myself with a witticism of enormous proportion - ho! ho! ho! And because the penny drops fairly quickly, we all have a good laugh.

I have used this so often, that this week, when trying it yet again, I felt a pang of guilt! Do I repeat myself so frequently in this way that I stand the chance of not only boring myself, but the clients as well?

As an active response, I began to assess each consultation, with a view to identifying cliches and repetitions according to 'Mr Roe the vet'... I was rapidly repaid with the painful truth!

My wife advised me of the frequency with which I enjoy my own little jokes, while my children pointed out that I say "realistically" far too often when speaking to clients, as well as requesting, "Give us a kiss for Christmas" from every dog showing willing during examination, adding that, "If I had a pound for every time..." is a comprehensive and dramatic way in which I make my points far too often.

Calling many pets, old scrap, wee squash, little chunker, little beanie and sausage, all showed up without fail and, to cap it all, I found myself referring to one small labrador puppy as a 'squashy binzo'

The dilemma worsened when one client looked vacantly at me when I described her cat as a 'short-wheel-based version!' Now I know that all you readers will understand that this refers to a chunky form of something, akin to the short and long wheel base versions of the very famous Land Rover four wheel drive, but on reflection, how on earth can I honestly expect a client to understand such strange descriptive terminology?

The answer is clear! I live gladly with the knowledge that my partial or complete eccentricity is tolerated, and even gladly accepted as normal or quite endearing by my clients. They do not appear to go around reporting the unusual 'gobblydegook' that emanates from my administrations, and I have the complete reason for my safety from the men in white coats because I reckon that my clients say exactly the same type of things which I do to their own pets - but safely within the confines of their own homes! Eric used to get away with it! Why can't I? I rest my case!

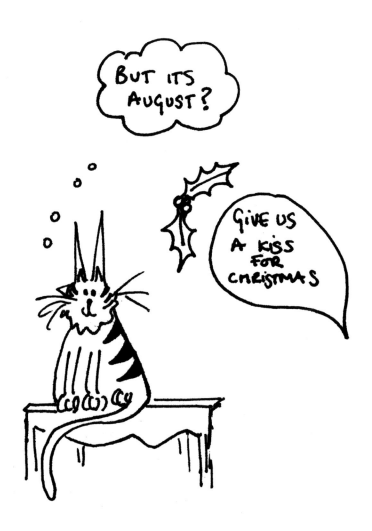

The colours of an operation? Red, Amber, then Green

Do I ever 'witter on' too much about my unadulterated respect for the ability of our pets to survive the most horrendous injuries, and undergo the most dramatic surgery, with a painful and prolonged recovery, yet still retain their trust in humans... Do I?

'No!' I hear you all cry. Good! Because the following story about a little cat called Amber, is quite literally the most amazing testament to nature that I have encountered in many a year.

Amber came in on a recent Saturday afternoon, with a report of lethargy and diarrhoea. I thought something was amiss, because she seemed very bulbous and squashy down her left side, from chest to back legs, and she was breathing rather heavily.

An x-ray confirmed my very worst fears. The bulbous, squashy bits were composed of internal organs, outside the chest wall, while other parts were up inside the chest cavity. It appeared that Amber was very seriously injured, with a ruptured diaphragm and possibly a ruptured chest or abdominal wall, which I suspected could only be caused by a car running a wheel completely over her little body. She had literally popped like a cork.

I had only one option. To attempt emergency surgery, immediately - and my goodness... It was dramatic!

Amber had a ruptured diaphragm, which means that as I was operating, I could see her heart beating through a hole between her chest and abdomen. Her poor little liver looked as if it had been smashed several times with a hammer, while her kidneys were severely bruised. Added to which, there was a four-inch tear in her abdominal wall, and a hole over her ribs, into which I could insert a fist. In essence, her whole, small body had been traumatised beyond belief.

The operation was a success. Nearly three hours of careful suturing and repair, with virtually constant administration of drip fed fluid, and drugs to control all manner of possible complications.

Even after the operation, and seventy four sutures, it was no more than a 'fifty-fifty' chance. She was desperately ill for seven days; unable to feed herself, but constantly buoyed up with regular visits from her devoted owners. She required injections every eight hours or so, to control pain and possible infection. She see-sawed between life and death, until Monday of this week, when, nine days after the massive operation, she gave me the sign that she would survive.

It went like this! She took a little bit of hand-fed food from my hand; stood up and used her litter tray, then groomed tentatively for about thirty seconds, before bumping heads with me and settling down to sleep. Normal cat service had returned. Now I knew that she would make it.

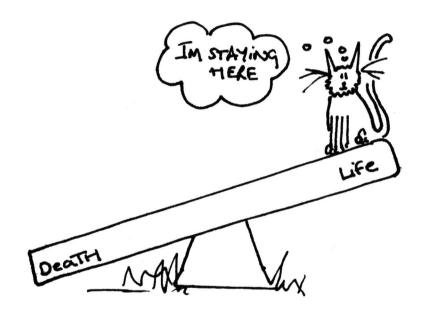

Something exotic for the weekend

This week. On Thursday to be precise, I was operating on a guinea-pig called Tufty, to remove a very unpleasant growth from the side of his face.

I started to think about how often vets carry out procedures on exotic species nowadays, compared to twenty years or so ago, when I first began to practise. You would see the odd rabbit, guinea-pig or rat, but not as frequently as we do today.

On this particular Thursday, I had a guinea-pig, rabbit and gerbil all undergoing surgery. A tortoise was in the hospital vivarium, being treated for anorexia, following waking too early from hibernation, and an iguana was arriving later for an x-ray of a suspected broken leg.

As I said, such days of 'exotic' consultation and surgery are becoming common-place, and generally more frequent. There are now several veterinary practices in Britain, which specialise in treating and accepting second opinion cases for our profession.

The Concise Oxford Dictionary defines exotic as: introduced from abroad; strange, bizarre, attractively strange or unusual, which only describes some of those species with which we deal under that umbrella-heading.

Having seen some of the vets who run these specialised practices, I feel 'exotic' is a wonderful term to apply to them in some cases. One was wearing bright blue operating clothes absolutely covered in prints of the species which he treats... snakes! The Christmas tree effect was truly bizarre, attractively strange, and unusual!

With the obvious growth in the interest in keeping more unusual species, vets must continue to keep abreast of all the new techniques and treatments, as well as dragging from the depths of our memory the myriad of anatomical variations and husbandry techniques specific to each type.

This is reason for my article this week? If you by any chance catch me on one of those days when I have had to spay a hamster; try to remember if it's the gerbil or chipmunk which has 31-32 day pregnancy; remove something from a snake's bottom, and help a pregnant terrapin to deliver its eggs via a caesarean section through its shell (which is mended with araldite and wire sutures), then please be very understanding! At my age, not only are the grey cells extended to their limits, trying to remember all those things, in terms of 'What's the answer?' and 'How do you do it?' But it's also difficult to cope with all that exotica. My wife tells me that it does my health no good at all!

127

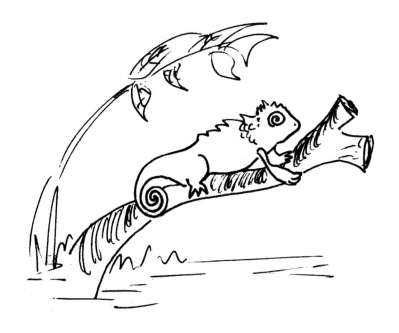

Perhaps this advice won't fall on deaf ears!

In November, I produced my definitive guide to 'the gentle art of pill popping' and I'm a little suspicious that far too few of my clients were paying the appropriate level of attention! In fact it seems quite clear that the numbers of cats that I am asked to attempt to dose with a pill is on the rise, and at quite an alarming pace.

Should any readers feel gently chided... fear not! I have such confidence in you that I am going to lead on to phase two of my cat husbandry and handling course.

Part two involves some advice on the vagaries of getting your cat into and out of that infernal basket, and involves some very basic techniques which might improve your success.

At the point of retrieving the basket from the dusty corner in the garage make a lot of comments about how strange it is to see woodworm in the wickerwork or airily muse about why mice should choose to place their droppings all over it. Even express surprise that a pigeon may have picked the lock and roosted all over it. On no account suggest that this has anything to do with Kitty. Even place it in the boot-sale pile if necessary

Lie about the time of the appointment! Pretend after the vet has put the phone down, 'Oh! That's six-o-clock then'... don't tell the truth about it being ten in the morning. Kitty knows just when to disappear.

Do not, on any account, put something nice in the basket in preparation for the scrummage. Biscuits, bits of ham, chicken or a favourite toy do not live in there. Kitty will note this from the shop round the corner, five hundred yards away, two hours before you have even thought about it. It spells 'nasty things'

Shut everything - every exit point, your bank account, and cancel the milk, and holidays. If it's warm outside, put the heating on at full blast. This may induce Kitty to think it's winter and fall asleep on the boiler, when you make the grab. Attach electrodes to Kitty to assess when REM (rapid eye movement) sleep, which is the deepest sleep state, is occurring.

Immediately smother all four legs and keep well away from the teeth. Do not feel confident that the tetanus jab and antibiotic cover collected yesterday will protect from all eventualities, so make sure that a list of all emergency services are close to hand. Four neighbours all holding a leg may just give you the edge! Do not trust gravity! Kitty can levitate out of a basket and manipulate any limb through any of the angle of a full circle. And never use a thick blanket or towel to plug Kitty into the small space. You will probably end up presenting me with a blanket/towel to vaccinate, surprised that Kitty isn't actually in there.

Also spend twenty five pence on two new buckles for the basket:- that single piece of string has had its day.

Express total amazement that Kitty refuses to come out of basket at the surgery: a car journey while crammed into a cubic foot; sniffed at, barked at while dumped on the clinic floor; the smell of weird chemicals; then some weird bloke grabbing at ones scruff, dragging one relentlessly into a phobic room for some torturous procedure!... bliss!

Be totally wowed that Kitty slinks, without fuss, back into the Abyss, with alacrity, after said procedure.

'Don't be concerned,' I usually reply, 'I don't take it personally!'

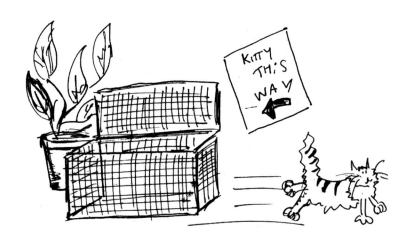

A small dog's rock-like determination to survive

Pete – or Fluffy Pete, as he is affectionately known by everyone at the clinic, leads something of a charmed life, more in keeping with the regulation nine of our feline friends.

It all began back in the summer, two years ago. I will quote from his records, taken off my computer records: 'Not well, severe anterior abdominal pain. Admit for x-ray and work up.'

'Not well' was a bit of an understatement. He was incredibly ill. His spleen was ten times its normal size; full of cancer, and requiring immediate surgical removal, which he survived with his normal alacrity. He was far more concerned with getting home to his doting owners after the surgery than convalescing sensibly.

But he made it through all his pain and suffering and, apart from a few niggling skin problems, he kept wonderfully well - until May of this year, when he came in again with a horribly swollen, uncomfortable abdomen!

Surgery followed, and we found a gastric torsion (a swollen stomach which is twisted), and a complication from the previous operation, which needed more, incredibly tense surgery to remove a lobe of his liver, during which I used up a week's supply of adrenaline.

He survived again! But the 'bearded Rolf' would have been proud of my 'touch and go' warnings to Pete's worried owners. I felt that we might loose the little man at any point from a myriad of possible post-op complications: from acute blood loss to embolism.

Fluffy Pete was having none of it. He only managed to be poorly for one day after the operation, after which he stood at his kennel gate, looking wanly at me, wondering why he was being so cruelly treated. Surely we understood that he had to get home!

He spent three days with us in total. His return home was an event to behold, with me having kittens at his dancing antics of pleasure, and waiting for his stitches to give way. Yet he simply looks down his nose at our concern for his welfare.

You see, in his eyes, we had no understanding of the importance of being able to bounce around and, more significantly, to dig up moles (his favourite game), which he started to do as soon as he arrived home. Not for him was there any concern about not having a spleen and a large part of your liver – life goes on!

He stays well to this day, with no further problems, as yet! We still don't know exactly why we nicknamed him 'Fluffy' after his first visit, because he certainly isn't fluffy. Yet the name has stuck, just like my endearing respect for this tough little chap, who has 'bounce' going through him like a stick of rock.

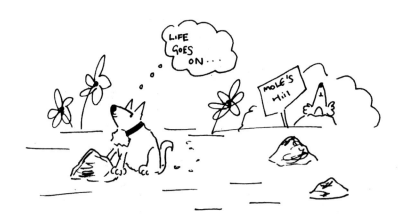

When 'not right' isn't left

There are times when being a vet is, to say the least, mysterious: by which I mean, it is sometimes difficult to find out what is going on with a pet that is not functioning correctly.

These are the moments when I wish clients would stop telling me so frequently that, 'You have to be cleverer than a doctor to be a vet, because the animals cannot tell you what is wrong!'

Perhaps this is true in some cases, but usually there is something which indicates where the illness is occurring and this, more often than not, is exemplified by that pet not doing its normal thing, so owners tell me that they are not right - and here I mean the pet, not the owner.

Genghis Chettleburgh, Cleo Hannant and Nobby Curtis are not characters from a Dickensian novel, but were cats who all appeared at the clinic this week, and were 'Not Right' (remember please, the eight letters available on my computer screen giving me a description of the problem my next patient is suffering from- according to our client!)

In all cases, the owner felt that their cats were off their food and miserable, with no idea why! And in every case, it was because those cats were suffering from a nasty disease which affects their mouths, essentially causing chronic ulceration of the membranes along the edge of the teeth and towards the back of the jaw, which is called gingivitis/stomatitis complex. It is complex, because nobody really knows why it occurs – lots of theories, but no certain answers! And it causes many cats to be 'Not Right', and frequently, you cannot stop it. Treatment controls the pain and swelling, but it comes back again, with vengeance, time and time again.

Now, it is worth me telling you that this tricky disease is only seen in this form in the domestic cat and, having monitored as many sufferers as I could, I have frequently seen a situation where it clears up completely, virtually overnight, when a stressful relationship between two or more cats ends, perhaps sadly, with the demise of the dominant one.

So are we seeing a condition in the cat which might be associated with stress? I don't know, and I probably won't be able to prove it. But ask yourself , how often we blame our illnesses upon our lifestyle? It may only be part of the story, but we must consider this when the holistic approach to all forms of medicine is becoming more appreciated.

My wife was 'Not Right' this week when Guinness, our tough, bruiser of a cat didn't turn up at his allotted time. She was worried, as ever, as to whether something awful had happened!

An hour later, she announced that all was well and, I quote, 'I knew he had come in, because I heard him playing the piano!'

Guinness cannot play the piano! – he simply enjoys walking along the keyboard when he comes into the house, with no particular tune in mind.

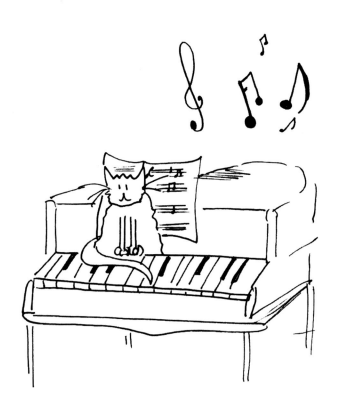

More advice on the art of being difficult

Dogs have nothing on us cats when it comes to being feisty! We know more than a thing or two when it comes to avoiding the vet, because vets should be avoided at all costs!

I have been thinking all week about how we beat them, after 'his' last article, telling us how well canines do it. Well they have it easy, considering that we are jammed into a basket, and left on the floor, being stared at, sniffed, and talked about; all before being whisked into the surgery to be prodded and jabbed by those people our owners call uncle, auntie or your doctor.

We are already captive, but don't let that get you down! Here are a few of the ways you can be difficult between the basket and leaving.

Always sit with your bottom facing the basket door. They have to reach in and turn you round to get you out, which can be very difficult, and might just allow you to sink a well-aimed fang into his hand.

But if he manages to turn you round successfully, then plant feet either side of the cage entrance - so as he pulls, you can resist and drag yourself back in. Remember, he's only got two hands; you've got four feet, which leaves at least a couple free to use those claws up his arm as you are unpleasantly extracted!

On occasions, he might try to tip you out of the box. You'll know this when he witters on about being like 'a cork in a bottle'. You just hold on to blanket, towel or basket edges to try and stay in there.

If this doesn't work, and you are ejected, then start complaining straight away. Any vet keeps a consultation short if you really make a fuss, with excuses like 'Oh he's really getting upset, let's not prolong this for too long.'… What rubbish! He's a wimp, who can't face a decent scrap!

Next, a few curdling yowls, flicking your tail and laying your ears flat – things which usually upset other cats by the way. Nothing like it to make it quick.

Finally, slide around the exam table. Slip off it, if you can, and make for the smallest space in the room. That usually gets you back into the basket pretty swiftly. If you've been really troublesome, you might get away without an injection. He'll give your human some tablets, and you know they can't give them to you unless they're hidden in something superbly tasty. I suppose that's some consolation.

So remember your CAT rules for visiting the vet: complain, aim, then scratch.

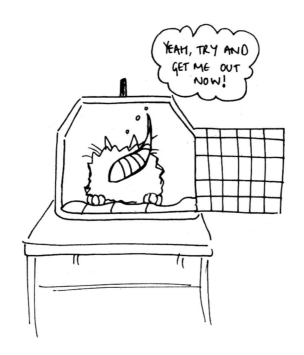

Can we have our ball back?

Forget about all those dreadful summer diseases and parasites which affect our pets at this time of the year, because I want to warn you about another danger that lurks in the background! The dastardly danger of playing ball with your pet.

Before continuing, I must just slip in a comment about the pleasure that I take in the warm appreciation shown by readers of this column. One client was so entranced by a recent missive that he was driven to applaud my efforts with, "I love your column each week. It really gives me and my wife so much pleasure. I don't know how you manage to make up those stories each week."… I smiled wanly.

For that particular client and, of course, everyone else, here is another story that I made up this week!

Bengi was on holiday on the Norfolk Broads, but had come with his mum and dad to visit the Norwich Sports Village, where youngest son of the family had started to play ball with him in a quiet corner of the carpark.

Ten minutes later, he was at the clinic, shaking his head from side to side, making a very strange noise, while trying to breath; and unusually, I'm sure that I kept hearing a bell tinkling!

Poor Bengi was really struggling, rocking from side to side, drawing in breath, looking as if he would collapse at any minute.

Mum and dad were at a loss to explain the events that had lead to this. Small child kept crying, saying "It wasn't me!"

I ascertained that small child had been left with the dog in the car while mum and dad dropped in to get a price list from the reception, but little more… I was still sure that I could still hear a bell tinkling, as Bengi shook his head!!

I had to move quickly. The little dog was beginning to loose consciousness! So he was rapidly anaesthetised - I opened his mouth to investigate.

Something blue and knobbly sat plum in the middle of his throat! I grabbed at it with a large pair of forceps and pulled out a blue, pimpled ball with a hole through the middle, and a bell that jangled in the hollow centre.

I'm convinced that the only thing that saved Bengi's life was the hole through the middle of the ball, allowing enough air through to keep him alive for a short period.

Small boy cried even more vehemently, "It wasn't me!" Bengi rapidly returned to normal, and was re-united with grateful mum and dad.

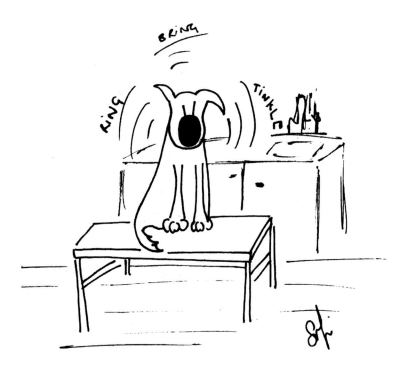

Always try to give the right advice

Staying healthy can be complicated - even for pets. We provide what we consider to be good nutrition and a healthy diet to our pets, but our animals, like humans, are consuming less fresh foods, more additives, and a smaller amount of natural sources of nutrients than ever before.

I hold a strong belief that advice in all these areas should be gently persuasive, rather than a sledgehammer.

With this in mind, I set about some serious education this week, in an attempt to bring the whole subject of pet health, diet, exercise and general well-being to the attention of as many clients as possible - it was my soapbox of the week, if you like.

My first effort was with a delightful old staffordshire bull terrier, called Archie, who, at twelve years old is rather arthritic, a little short of breath, and selectively deaf.

'What do you feed him? I asked.

'Anything he likes! He's partial to a bit of Chinese takeaway or Indian, but what he enjoys best is the fat I cut off the joint at the weekend.'

I was determined to advise, 'What about his exercise?'

'He doesn't like that much! I take him in the car down to the woods, let him out, and sometimes have a bit of snooze myself. By the time I wake up he's sometimes back in the car, sleeping himself. As I said, he doesn't like rushing round too much.

I abandoned my lost cause and, with stealth, approached a client a little later during surgery. They had brought along an obese cat, probably five kilos overweight (twice it's acceptable size), and I was convinced that I could bring my enigmatic charm to bear, and succeed in improving this little cat's lot.

'He's a bit chunky,' I began, smiling benevolently.

'Is he?' The owners just looked at me.

'Well, he might benefit from some weight loss. It would make him more mobile and perhaps prevent heart problems and possibly diabetes developing in later life. Also remember that arthritis is far more likely in overweight cats!'

Next came the 'coup de grace' : the comment that stumped me totally.

'He was born big! Anyway, we like him big. He's not happy unless he can keep eating. He eats two tins a day, and we get it down the cash and carry.'

So as I was saying. Keep a good eye on your pet's health and try to ignore advice from me, especially when it might spoil your pet's enjoyment of life!

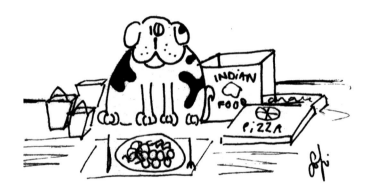

A Rotten start for Jackson

Jackson, a quiet, easy-going labrador, and his owners didn't know what they had let themselves in for - nor did I!

Getting their head round the fact that he had the most aggressive form of a widespread lymphatic cancer, with the shortest life expectancy of perhaps six months, was painful enough. But then to have to decide whether to treat him, with all the potential anti-cancer drug side effects, but the hope of remission, or to entrust him to the vagaries of nature, compounded their suffering.

We talked and talked, hoping for the right choice. We even asked Jackson what he felt. And a week later it was mutually decided that we would begin the chemotherapy of weekly intravenous drugs and divided doses of oral drugs.

That first treatment was a revelation. Jackson returned pretty much to his old self, demanding his usually walks; the lethargy of the previous weeks replaced as the drugs rapidly got to work. Even though he'd seemed a little wobbly afterwards, this soon subsided.

I was happy - the owners delighted! As their dog seemed to get back his old sparkle.

He bounced in for his second weekly injection. All went well. We really thought we had begun to fight the disease.

Then catastrophe! As day by day, nearly every unpleasant side effect and symptom possible from the drugs reared its ugly head.

First he became disorientated, then weak in all his limbs. He began to vomit, and a raging gut upset followed, causing his owners to wonder whether this might be the end for him.

This all went on for a week. I felt so responsible, but so helpless because there was so little that could be done to reverse these horrible signs.

Jackson himself seemed to be fighting gamely - holding his own, but eventually had to be hospitalised, with tubes and pipes everywhere, giving him the vital fluids and nutrition without which he wouldn't survive. Even then, he still had a look as if he had one final big effort inside him.

He was allowed home for the weekend, but was back in for a further observation and treatment regime midweek; finally beginning to turn the corner on Friday, looking a little stronger, eating well and, most importantly, showing that he was still determined to make it a little way down the road for a walk.

His symptoms should abate, and luckily, the remission from the first drug doses has prevailed - but now another decision has to be made regarding what we do next. If the drugs cause him this much illness, is it really worth continuing? The answer is that we cannot tell, but drug type and doses will have to change if we do continue, because we cannot let him suffer again like he has these last two weeks.

Yet one thing is sure. That Jackson will still be at the family meeting to try to make the right choice.

141

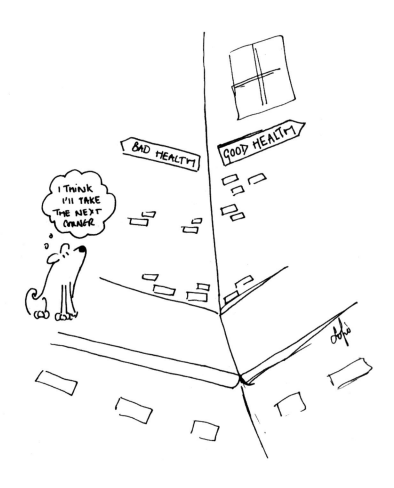

A rather dangerous length of string

Sophie, a little cat just under a year old was losing weight, and looked rather thin and poorly for one so young: yet for a cat who had been vomiting for some while that, perhaps, was not unusual.

What was strange included regular stomach swelling, increased desire to drink, and a penchant for chomping on inordinate amounts of grass.

All this went on for several weeks. She improved on drugs which settled her stomach and decreased her desire to vomit, but still she deteriorated until it was decided that we had to search more deeply for the answers.

An x-ray revealed strange densities in her stomach and an unusual thickening lower into the bowel.

We had to operate immediately, in an attempt to find out what these strange masses were.

I looked in the stomach initially and found a huge mass of hair, grass and fibrous material constricting a couple of pieces of what seemed to be chicken bone, with a piece of thin string winging its way down into the depths of the intestine.

The chase continued! A foot or two later, further down, I found the second identified mass of bone, with a very thick, tenacious covering of something rather high smelling and unpleasant, connected by the first identified piece of string, which passed through this mass off into the further reaches of the gut! – where would it end?

I followed the taut feeling down to a point where the intestine was scrunched up into a concertina-shape by the continuing string and something holding it tight a little further beyond, which appeared to be another piece of bone, but the tight string had cut through the wall of the intestine (rather like a cheese wire), around which the tissues had healed, catching it up even more firmly at this point.

How this string had got to where it was, in quite this manner, was an absolute mystery; and quite how this little cat had survived without a complicating infection or severe blood loss, I cannot say. It seems miraculous that she could feed, do her ones and twos, and function reasonably well while all this trauma was occurring inside.

But she's not out of the woods yet! She needs to heal those four operation points in her intestine, and the point at which I had to reconstruct the wall of her intestine due to the damage caused by the string. So there's a long way to go! Yet she showed her true mettle very rapidly after such major surgery by nearly having a 'dicky fit' when we fed another cat in the nextdoor kennel and left her bowl empty.

Sophie demanded feeding, just twelve hours post-operatively, even though it said 'Nil by mouth' on her hospital sheet. Just a little liquid convalescent diet was given, which she engulfed, proving just how little she thought of her ordeal.

This episode clearly shows us how silly our pets can be with the things they try to swallow, and how a length of string can result in the need for very invasive surgery and intensive care! Cross all your fingers with me for a successful recovery of little Sophie.

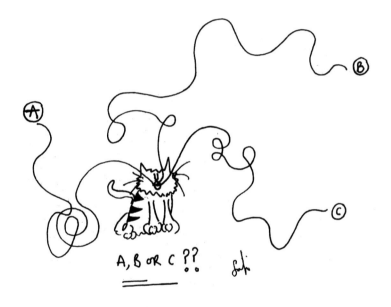

A, B OR C ??

A nifty haircut for Mable

I couldn't decide who looked or felt worse: Mable the cat or her owner, in as much that both were suffering dreadfully. The little cat as a result of a hefty blow from a car in a road traffic accident. Her owner from the trauma of seeing a much-loved pet in such distress.

Poor Mable! A fractured lower jaw, fractured hard palate (roof of her mouth), severe damage and bleeding in her right eye, and contusions and bruising around the head, with a nasty concussion – she was in a poor state!

Thankfully, some powerful pain and shock relief therapy provided her with a comfortable night, but then it was down to the serious stuff of repairing her severe injuries, and contemplating her future requirements to enable maintenance of feeding i.e. keeping her alive.

Some careful surgery to correct her facial injuries, involving wires and various implants returned her to something akin to a normal looking cat, but she was so badly bruised and so sore that the only way to feed her was via a thing called a nasogastric tube: a rubber tube going down her nose and into her stomach, by-passing her mouth.

Now I've had one of these doing the same thing, and it's horrible! And I'm sure that Mable felt the same thing - but it had to be done.

I was on call over the weekend, during which my daughters and I regularly had to feed Mable via this tube with a specialist, concentrated liquid feed – and she hated that. In fact she was very depressed through this whole period, not helped by the fact that she had to have all the hair from her face, including whiskers, shaved for her operation (which I'm sure made her feel very self-conscious). She did look rather strange with her little skinny head popping out from a very large, hairy body.

By late Sunday evening, as luck would have it, the severely traumatised nasogastric tube gave up! Breaking just at the point joining with the feeding connector, leaving no option but to remove it.

Mable immediately blossomed, rubbing her less painful head against us, the bars of her cage and anything else in sight. She started calling to us, chirruping and generally socialising as if a huge weight had been lifted off her shoulders. It was remarkable as much as a joy to see this transformation, which has continued with careful convalescence and help in feeding from her owner over the past week to the position where, despite my advice to the contrary, she is eating the other cat's solid food, and generally acting in a very normal Mable-like manner - but she got some way to go before full recovery: her jaw and a few slightly-misplaced teeth will require a bit more surgical attention, but then what's that for tough cat like Mable, when compared to the dodgy haircut.

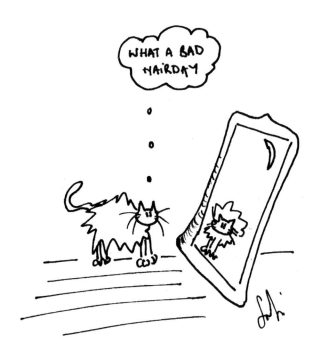

Pet owners watching the box

It came home to me this week, that I am no longer the expert that I presume to be! A delightful owner announced, during a consultation, that she suspected her cat was suffering from 'a bacterial-viral disease'.

I have a problem in that I cannot hide what I am thinking - my face generally gives the game away. Thus, I burst into laughter, and then back-peddled rapidly to appease the dear lady, whose opinion I had scoffed so lightly.

'You generally have to have one or the other. It's unlikely to be both together,' I said gently, and with a tinge of generosity.

She still seemed confused, so I went on to talk about how easy it is to watch the multitude of vet programmes on the telly, and pick up the wrong end of the stick about disease processes… she was still confused!

I eventually just blamed Rolf, of the Harris variety, and smoothed this chat to a conclusion - and Rolf certainly must take some of the blame! Not only has he provided the discerning public with masses of new information about pets and vets, but frequently, just as I sit down to supper, after a busy day at the office, who should appear on the box but himself, offering, "Did you see that?" or "It was touch and go" in his inimitable Aussie tones.

Now it isn't because I dislike him or the other vet shows that have spawned from the marvellous Animal Hospital, but it is because it forces me to give my opinion, 'Oh dear!' I start, 'He should have done it that way' or (sharp intake of breath), 'I wouldn't do it that way.'

You see, armchair expertise rules. And I am guilty! But the shock-waves reverberate far and wide. The power of the television has begun to influence those things that clients request as treatments.

It was not until this year that we regularly began to spay pet rabbits, usually to try to effect a change in aggressive behaviour or womb problems. I spayed two this week, which is quite unusual, considering that I gave no advice to try this operation - it must have come from the television vets.

Likewise, it was not until Vet's in Practice, that the idea of removing maloccluding front teeth of rabbits permanently was requested. We usually clip them regularly, but now this new operation will take hold, I'm sure! It seems that a lot of techniques for medical and surgical practices on more exotic species are finding favour because of televisual exposure - which is really exciting!

So the power of our televisions rules, Ok! But not in the case of a dear old gentleman, who requested me to spay his gill ferret this week.

"I suppose you saw that on the television," I smiled back at him.

"Narrgh," he replied.

"Oh! I'm surprised," I countered.

"Why should you be! I ain't got a telly!

147

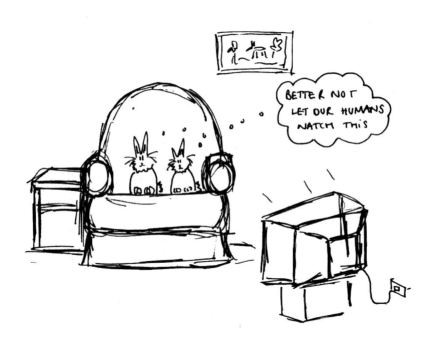

A little help with the decorating

The endless decorating has begun again at the practice. I can relax about the person doing the job because (most importantly) it's not me and, secondly, our decorator is a real gem, fitting in with our requirements by working late into the night and at weekends.

Yet this does not prevent certain levels of upheaval! This week it was the turn of the kennel block floor to receive a spruce up - which might not sound too taxing. But it means complete mayhem, because we can't keep any animals in their normal kennels due to the fumes as the paint cures, and it cannot be tramped upon for six hours after application.

I know this sounds like the advice on the back of a paint tin but it sets the scene for what happened next, in as much as I had to cram all the patients who were staying over the weekend into a small room in their individual mobile kennels which meant that they could all communicate with each other and concoct mischief for me. I should have realised that it was going to be similar to controlling a bunch of unruly fourth formers!

It seemed that those cats were determined to tip over as many water bowls as possible; push little bits of food through the bars onto the floor, and fill as many litter trays as 'humanly' possible, meaning copious amounts of unpleasant things to clear up, when everything to do it with was in the wrong place or required a long trip round the outside of the practice to get it.

Breagha, a little tortoiseshell won the litter tray stakes, filling a mighty nine trays, while Betty managed to tip over her water bowl whenever I turned my back. Boots was little better, but his emptying was acceptable: being diabetic, he was drinking excessively and drained every fresh bowl within a couple of minutes.

Sara just sat in her cage hissing at me as I performed my regular Mrs Mop performance, and Travis (Dear Travis of previous article fame) continued to try and pick my pockets whenever I stood near his cage. He has pretty much fully recovered and has just won the practice award for the most endearing feline head tilt of the year.

Yet all of this was surpassed by Shearer, a small black and white cat who suffered a nasty fracture of the femur, repaired on Saturday afternoon, after which he progressed so well that he was standing and mobile by Sunday morning. All was going well until I turned round to check that he had eaten his breakfast on that morning to find (after a double take) his cage empty. The funniest part of this was realizing how foolish it was of me to lift his perfectly flat bedding to see if he was hiding underneath.

I searched the practice in mild panic and eventually found one Shearer sitting comfortably on the x-ray table in the x-ray room licking his front paws with great pleasure, minus a carefully placed leg support which had been immobilising his leg.

He seemed no worse for his ordeal and I realised that he had triumphantly noticed that the catch on his cage door was not properly holding and made his escape.

The kennel block floor looks lovely but I'm only just coming down from the stress of it all.

149

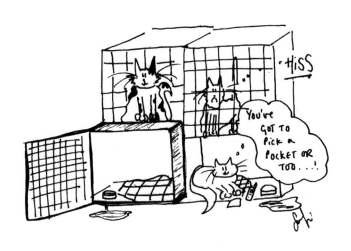

The Pleasure and pain of a vet's life

I am a lucky chap! Throughout my career as a vet, I have had the most marvellous experiences.

Treating famous horses such as Mill Reef, Grundy and Star Appeal at the National stud is fondly remembered, while helping the remarkable Derby winning greyhound, Westpark Mustard, through a severe leg injury gave me great pleasure. And successfully healing any injured animal, even without a famous name, gives huge satisfaction, every time.

In essence, being a vet can give you the most marvellous quality of life, and provide you with some wonderful experiences but, like most professions, while learning, there is no gain without some pain, and I certainly had many painful episodes along the way.

As a student, and being expendable, I was regularly caused suffering, from being the chosen one to take a dog out into the rain to collect a urine sample in a soggy kidney dish (which often ended up as more rain than urine) or to hold a limb out of the way during an operation, until total numbness set in. It was meant to be painful! It was expected.

But most dramatic of these regular events, occurred during an operation on a hereford bull, with an interdigital cyst: a common problem, treated frequently twenty years ago with cryosurgery - a technique using liquid nitrogen to freeze the tissues.

I was sitting on the bull's neck, holding the tank full of liquid nitrogen when it decided to stand up, instead of remaining sedated, lifting me and my tank of precious, very cold fluid into the air. I held on for a grim death, as the animal started to trot around its stable.

The rest of the students, and the surgery lecturer (who shall remain nameless, but is today a very famous expert in our profession) legged it, leaving me to continue the rodeo performance.

I will never forget the lecturer shouting out compassionately, as I held on, 'For God's sake save the b——y machine, Tim. It's worth six hundred pounds'. Of course, I could just take care of myself! How I presumed that I could save the machine and wrestle a ton of staggering bull to the floor defies common sense, but after about six circuits of the stable, he simply collapsed into the deep bed of straw and sat there, looking bemused. I received a deserved ovation, while the smiling lecturer retrieved his precious machine from my grasp.

But I got him back!... A few months later, after numerous complaints from aforementioned lecturer about the scruffy male students not wearing ties, we decided to 'toe the line' at our mare pregnancy diagnosis class.

We all arrived, very professionally attired, in our standard issue, waterproof calving gowns and green wellies, wearing the largest and gaudiest bow ties that we could muster. Mine measured nine inches across and was deep velvet-blue, adorned with delicate pink dots! 'I suppose you think that's funny?' he retorted... We did!

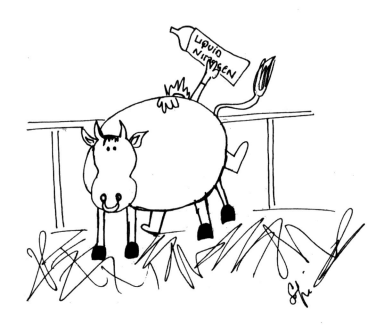

152

I'm always telling you that, 'You won't believe what happened today?'

The sun has been shining today! I thought an article about 'Summer problems for pets' might be appropriate, but then, Fluffy Pete, a remarkable little crossbred dog, who has survived another episode of tough surgery must deserve a mention at some point!

Then it happened!… What? I hear you all say, with baited breath.

What happened was morning surgery, which tumbled along with one incredibly unusual event after another.

It began while I was vaccinating Mrs Butler's three cats. In passing, she mentioned that one of them had acquired a little visitor in the form of a tick, attached to the top of his head. She then revealed her marvellous remedy for said 'beasties', obviously passed down from an old sage of yesteryear.

'Someone told me to put neat gin on it,' she rejoiced, 'But my daughter said brandy was better!'

I was wonderfully bereft of an answer to that. We laughed about the possibilities of such therapy, then proceeded to check all three cats: the last of which she reported as the shy, retiring member of the family, who has the unfortunate habit of inappropriate urination in the house, probably because of feelings of insecurity - but Mrs Butler hadn't finished.

She reported that he took greatest pleasure in piddling over the telephone.

And that when she took her malfunctioning camera to be mended, she was advised that it was full of 'fluid material' of some form, by Dr Camera! This brings a whole new meaning to territory marking.

It took me a few consults to stop tittering about the Butler family, but this quickly turned to incredulity when a small, fourteen year old persian cat arrived for a check up. Her owner told me that she had just arrived back home, after being lost, and that she had noticed her sitting in her neighbour's garden.

'How long has she been away,' I asked.

'One and a half years,' she replied… I was almost speechless.

We mused over the possibilities, but finally, having checked that she was indeed the very cat, lost so long ago, via her identichip implant, we decided that it was simply a wonderful event, only matched by the return of Frank Butcher to Eastenders

This was a particularly apt comment, because the little tibetan terrier which came in afterwards, just happens to be the very same TV star dog which Ethel rescued in Albert square, several years ago, feeding it a meat pie and taking it to a rescue centre.

She also appears on the front of the RSPCA nationwide neutering brochure, alongside her daughter's tabby cat.

I felt honoured to be treating such a little star. She's a little frail now, with quite severe eye disease, but she still has that aura of fame!

What a morning, I thought: the events of which had delighted, amazed and impressed, all within one hour. Summer advice and my little friend, Fluffy Pete, will just have to wait.

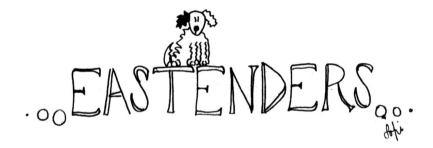

Caring for an 'Array' of hedgehogs

Did you know that a group of hedgehogs is called an Array ?

Well over Christmas and New Year I was party to such an Array – several people brought in hedgehogs which they had been feeding regularly in their gardens during the late autumn and early winter: most of them suffering from respiratory illnesses. I'm sure brought on by the stress of late breeding due to a mild year and a sudden cold snap, which young hoglets are unable to cope with after their protective parents have retired for the winter in deep undergrowth or the local compost heap.

A great friend of all 'spikeys', Mrs Lynn from Brundall, alerted me to the need for looking out for these hoglets all winter! You see hedgehogs tend to take periodic sleeps during the winter, so many who wake up during the toughest, coldest periods are, as a result, ravenous.

This is when we need to help them out in our gardens. So it seems valuable to give a little advice to those of you who are concerned for your local 'spikey'.

It's unlikely that you will come across a very young hoglet at this time of year, but adolescents may be wandering around looking for valuable calories.

Don't feed cow's milk at all! Goat's milk is fine. Try puppy or kitten food, bread mashed with gravy, scrambled egg and, if you're not squeamish, plain mealworms, earthworms and slugs. Peanuts, muesli, digestive biscuits and fruit are all much appreciated and even try a multivitamin, like Abidec drops as a supplement.

Look out for general health: snuffling with coughs and runny eyes and/or nose may suggest a lungworm infestation or chest infection, both of which require veterinary attention, as will chronic signs of diarrhoea.

(Sorry to get a little personal but do remember that normal young hedgehog number twos are a greeny-blue colour).

If the hedgehog appears to be heaving with ticks and fleas, then another visit to the vet will be required. These parasites treat the hedgehog like a hotel.

If you do need to rescue a hedgehog which seems unwell, check initially that it is not simply weak from cold or dehydration. Cold inhibits their desire to eat, if severe. So put them in a dry box with a 'hotty' wrapped in a dry towel. If that doesn't stimulate activity to feed and drink, look for some other reason such as fractures, infection and even heavy parasite burden. Also bear in mind the potential injury from toxic substances such as pesticides and creosote, commonly found languishing in the dark corners of the garden.

You can help the regular, healthy, visiting hoglet by creating a feeding station in the garden: a rectangular plastic tray, upturned and secured by bricks on top requires a four inch hole cut in one side. Food can be placed inside on shallow saucers. This allows them to feed safely, protected from the elements and inquisitive moggies. Don't put the water saucer in with the food! It might just end up tipped over or drown young hoglets caught in a confined space.

Happy hog-watching!

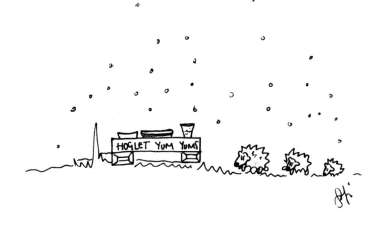

Cheek by jowl with Corfiot cats

Corfu, deliciously verdant and veiled with a tranquillity which only the likes of Gerald Durrell could capture in his book 'My family and other animals'; helped by picture postcard seaside villages like Koulara, where he lived as he wrote that book.

The Vetinary and his family are on their summer hols to the sun, where we always seem destined to suffuse our veterinary lives back home with the animal culture of our destination.

Invariably I received a list of 'is that cat limping' or 'Oh! poor thing. They obviously don't care about animals here!'

In fact I'm most concerned that if we reach home one day, post holiday, and my wife is missing, then she may have eventually transcended to the throne of slightly eccentric local cat lady - living a subsistence existence with a panoply of local feline strays saved from scratching out a life – ho hum!

Corfiotes are not like us about their pets. The lithe, stilt-legged, oriental-like collections of moggies attending waiter-like at the tables of the local tavernas, willing scraps from open air tables of restaurant revellers are testament to the disinformation about pet flea month and expensive television campaigns about parasite treatment; and their world-wariness typifies the 'Shoo', 'Don't feed the cats' mentality of the locals.

Don't get me wrong! I don't think cruelty is an issue, but they don't seem to care as much as back home, seemingly viewing people like me as a bit of an oddity.

But the slow pace of life does allow one to savour lots of little mental momentoes. For example, there are no cats-eyes marking the hillside, switchback roads, unless you count the live cats, sitting imperiously watching the world go by, late at night. One little cat was so enthralled with trying to catch a moth that a small traffic jam collected, while other jaywalkers threw inquisitorial glances when asked politely to move. Well that's cats for you!

'Don't feed the cats' was as a red rag to a bull to all of us. Each feline being scrutinised by the Griswalds for signs of ill-health as it was slipped a morsel or two.

My youngest daughter even demanded my intervention at one venue for a white cat being beaten by a merciless old woman!... Close scrutiny showing that she was in fact playing a game with it with her fly swatter.

Where could life be so laid back? That a litter of kittens would be allowed to tumble around a taverna, enjoying an endless game, as the parents, sitting graciously in a nearby olive tree keep watch. In typical fashion, our feline friends have colonised, and continue to utilize our human existence.

What a place to set up a veterinary practice, bringing our hi-tech, North-European skills and advice to a needy animal population. But, then again, hey-ho! It's siesta time - ice blue sky, quenching, poolside iced tea. I'll rest a little more before developing that idea. 'Laid back' must be catching.

Next week! continuing the holiday stories of 'Old Artha', bouncing pups and a mule with attitude.

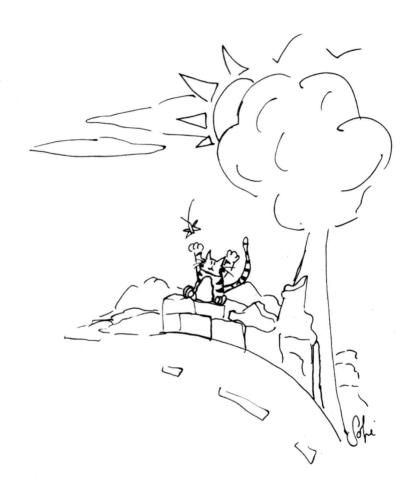

It's too late,
I've been 'pugged'

We have a saying in our family that saying No! is much more potent than Yes!, when making a decision. And it is strange, isn't it? That when there is a difference of opinion, when making a choice, the negative side usually wins.

So there I was surrounded by my 'Three Witches of Eastwick' i.e. wife and children, all of whom had spent the previous weeks trying as hard as they may to convince me of the value of adding a little black pug-dog to our menagerie.

The imminence of my youngest daughter's seventeenth birthday was prime argument, followed by, 'We'll look after him. You won't have to do anything! We will get up during the night and feed/change/water him dee-dum dee-dum..'

I held out on my side. My arguments against pugs which I mentioned in an earlier article were paraded professionally, and I thought I had won the day.

But last week a very calm (even calculating) wife gently tried again, and in a moment of quite surprising mellowness, I said that because we always tried to make decisions based on the majority opinion - and if they respected all my reasons for not having this puppy, then the decision was up to them (sounds really stuffy, doesn't it?). My wife did calmly announce that if we got the pug, then perhaps she would buy me the new digital camera I've been staring at longingly in the toyshop window.

Talk about speed! The girls flew into action and within hours the already sourced fourteen week old little chap was at home - 1.6 kilos of chunky, in your face, cheeky-chappy, who I fell totally in love with within minutes, even after this carefully planned Blitzkrieg.

His little goggly eyes, scrunched up nose and endearing personality have melted every heart, and I even ended up carrying him round the Dixon centre in Hellesdon, to choruses of every type of Ooo! And Ahh! imaginable.

He had twenty visitors at our 'Meet the baby Pug' party over the weekend. He behaved impeccably well in front of all his new aunts and uncles, and has had a constant flow of admirers ever since. In fact I'm feeling a little jealous.

It took no time to name him Louis, after the celebrated Mr Armstrong, with the little addition of something extra - so he's Louis-le-Pug (although Stinky-P has use to describe him frequently in the last few day), and he's living up to his pugnaciousness (he even toughed it out against the Dyson on Wednesday) with a confidence and joy of life which cause constant laughter.

But at the same time he's a really intelligent little chap, who seemingly knows just how to tease our other dogs, Pru and Wellie to within an inch of annoyance - their fluffy tails being a constant incitement to grab and pull.

He really is a lovely, adorable little chap (and I still stand by all my reasons which said no). In fact so lovely that I'm spending some time this week-end taking some 'puppy-pix' with my new digital camera.

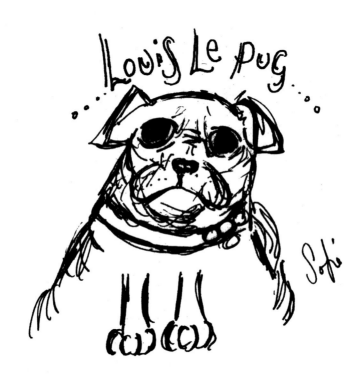

Tim has been a vet for over twenty years and continues to work in his own clinic close to Norwich, where he lives with his wife, two daughters, and an array of animals.

During this time he has appeared on Anglia Television and continues to write articles about his day to day life for local publications.

This book contains a small selection of those articles, in no particular order, which have been collected together in this first edition, supported by cartoons drawn by his daughter, Sophie.

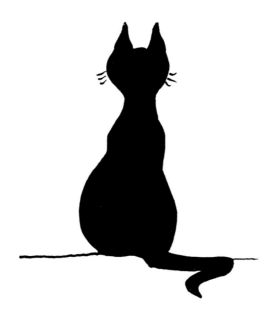